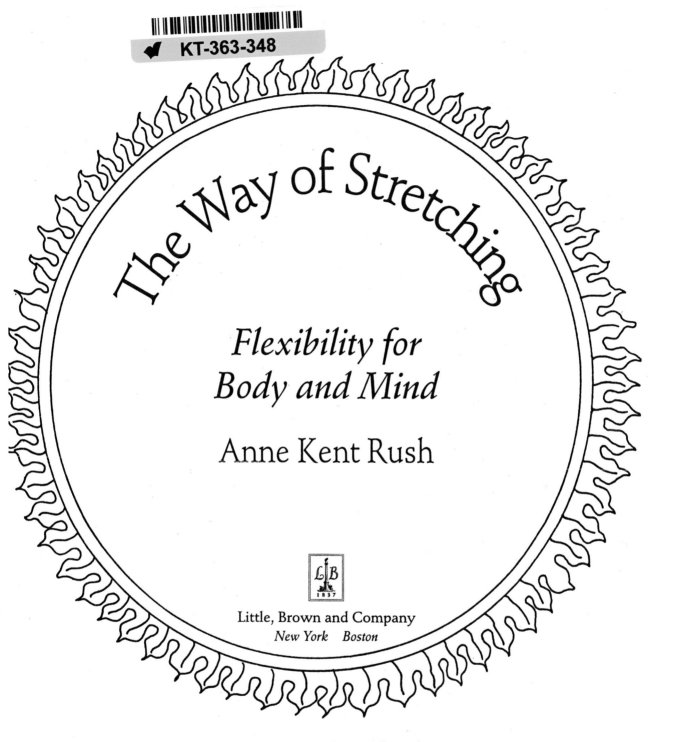

The Way of Stretching

Flexibility for Body and Mind

Anne Kent Rush

Little, Brown and Company

New York   Boston

Little, Brown and Company
Time Warner Book Group
1271 Avenue of the Americas, New York, NY 10020
Visit our Web site at www.twbookmark.com

First Edition: August 2005

The information herein is not intended to replace the services of a trained
health-care professional. You are advised to consult your health-care
professional with regard to matters relating to your health and, in particular,
in regard to matters that may require diagnosis or medical attention.

Library of Congress Cataloging-in-Publication Data

Rush, Anne Kent.
    The way of stretching : flexibility for body and mind /
    Anne Kent Rush. — 1st ed.
        p.   cm.
    ISBN 0-316-17231-6
    ISBN 978-0-316-17231-8

    1. Stretching exercises. 2. Meditation. 3. Chakras. I. Title.
RA781.63.R873 2005
613.7'1 — dc22   2005005740

10 9 8 7 6 5 4 3 2 1

Q-MB

Printed in the United States of America

Dedicated to
H. H. the Dalai Lama of Tibet
and his inspiration of courageous flexibility

OM MANI PADME HUM HRI

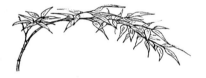

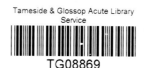
WB541
RUS
2005

Praise for
The Way of Stretching

"Anne K⟨
pr⟨

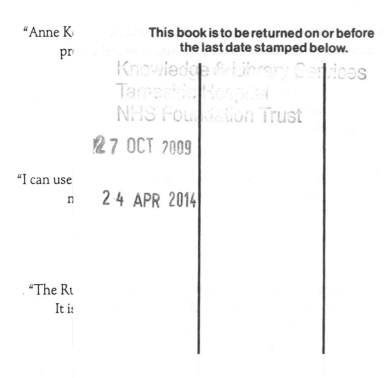
"I can use
n⟨

. "The R⟨
It i⟨

By Anne Kent Rush

The Amazing Grits Song Book

The Basic Back Book: The Complete Manual of Back Care

The Back Rub Book: How to Give and Receive Great Back Rubs

Classic Cameos and Incomparable Intaglios: Yesterday and Today

Feminism as Therapy (with Anica Vesel Mander)

Getting Clear: Body Work for Women

Greta Bear Goes to Yellowstone National Park

*Massage for Total Well-Being: Massage and Meditation for the
Seven Centers of Health*

The Modern Book of Massage: Five-Minute Vacations and Sensuous Escapes

The Modern Book of Yoga

The Modern Book of Stretching: Strength and Flexibility at Any Age

Moon, Moon: An Encyclopedia of Moon Lore and Goddess Mythology

The Omega Book of Bodywork Basics

Romantic Massage: Ten Unforgettable Massages for Special Occasions

The Way of Stretching: Flexibility for Body and Mind

CONTENTS

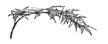

Part I   The Way of Stretching

Part II Flexibility Exercises

Part I

The Way of Stretching

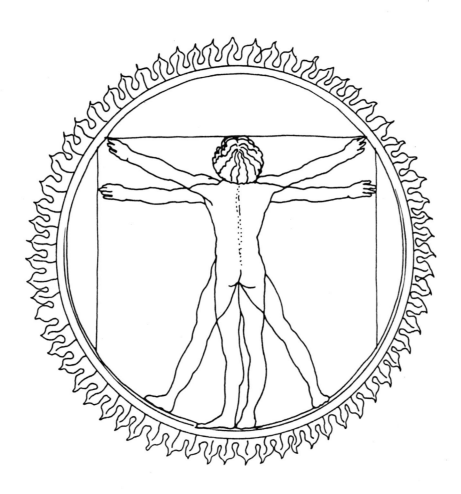

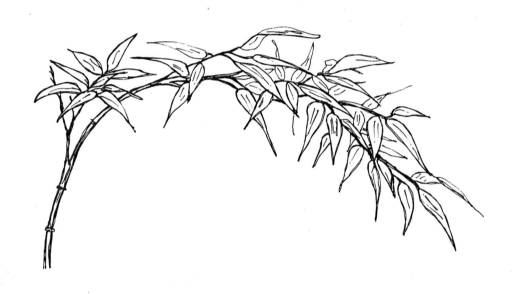

BODY STRETCHING

Very Good News

Proper stretching for maximum athletic condition involves many qualities that a couch potato would adore. Less is more. Each stretch works best if done only briefly, literally for two seconds. Easy does it. Nothing but a relaxed muscle will stretch. Pain is against the rules. Mental and physical comfort are required for top results. Slow down and smell the success. Periodic rests are necessary. It's a gymnastic that keeps on giving. After you're done, your increased circulation continues to flush toxins and spread oxygen and healing throughout your body. The only challenge to a couch potato is the necessity of being consistent with the gentle routines. However, this aspect is sweetened by the instant gratification a proper stretch delivers in the form of small waves of pleasure in your muscles. Begin a safe stretching program, and get ready to get hooked.

The Way of Stretching

Contrary to general practice, stretching is not merely a separate movement series done before and after exercise. Safe stretching is the blueprint for how to move your body at all times, during any activity, to achieve the most efficient, comfortable, powerful, and healing pattern of movement, and it includes mental exercise, too. As such, safe stretching is best done in brief interludes rather than as one long workout. Interspersing safe stretches during your exercise breaks, as well as during your daily work, gradually trains your body to perform proper motion patterns at all times and to release the strains that build up during the day. Consistent safe stretching ensures that your sport as well as your routine movement will soothe and renew rather than strain and exhaust you. An expanded, tailor-made, safe stretching program that includes strength building also can be developed as your complete daily exercise.

You already have all the muscle length you need. Controlling flexibility requires control of an autonomic (unconscious) function.

— Pavel Tsatsouline,
Russian flexibility expert

The Way of Stretching combines three approaches to integrate (1) exercise positions for toning the whole body, (2) breathing techniques for energy rejuvenation, and (3) mental development, including meditation and visualization. Uniting these techniques balances body, mind, and spirit — key to ongoing physical and mental flexibility.

The exercises in this book come from my many years of researching and writing about preventive health care and from the numerous training programs on psychology and exercise that I've taken and taught, from aikido to Zen. The stretches are designed to stimulate all the muscles and joints in your body, including your brain cells. The way in which you move is the key to how fully your mind and body benefit — and to how much fun you have as you go.

Safe Stretching

How we interpret the word "stretching" in our minds before we start to move alters how we perform. Many of us assume that stretching means extending our muscles as far as we possibly can, even if this hurts a bit, in order to increase range of movement. Actually, overextension shortens muscles, decreases range of motion, and sometimes injures the tissue. We need to use a new definition that explains stretching as a process of working muscles gently and fully to their limit but not beyond. This is what is meant by the phrase "safe stretching." To promote safe stretching as you exercise, it can be helpful to think of *lengthening* the muscle rather than stretching it.

Working within your muscle range is the main key to the remarkable limbering effects of properly performed exercise. We often resist practicing moderation. It's tempting to push our limits, because doing so seems to satisfy an urge for instant progress. But pushing too hard is a short-term high. When the morning after dawns, our muscles ache, shorten, cramp. We may have torn some tissue that will require several days of inactivity to allow healing. This is the "one step forward, two steps backward" approach to fitness. In the long run, if we stretch with impatient overextension of our muscles, we develop a strained body with minimum range and stiffness of movement. As we age, the overstretched, overstrained body will present many problems. Stretch in haste; repent at leisure.

Would you rather have instructions screamed harshly at you or explained gently? Most people respond better to being told something calmly and respectfully, and our muscles react the same way. Light, smooth movement creates less defensive backlash in a muscle, less shortening of tendons, and more healthy flexibility and graceful ease of movement than a forced, extreme stretch.

The facts about muscle functioning support my experience that gentle, slow exercise systems are the most effective in promoting health, strength, and flexibility. Yet, in spite of evidence to the contrary, many people are still attracted to rough, fast exercise routines. These satisfy a Western urge for the promise of quick solutions and reflect a persistent attitude that power can't be simple or gentle. In actuality, the most powerful concepts or programs are also often the simplest.

Many excellent low-impact exercise systems exist from which to choose. Some of my favorites that I have trained in, to varying degrees, are Active-Isolated Stretching, Alexander Technique, Aston-Pattering, Feldenkrais, Hatha Yoga, Proskauer Awareness, Rosen Method, Rubenfeld Synergy, and Trager Integration.

After thirty-five years experimenting with varieties of wonderful systems, I have formulated a new technique that I have named the Rush Reverse. A need exists for a simpler stretching system that does not require years of complex training, that can be combined with any other exercise system, that works right away, and that is based on the most recent scientific understanding of how safe stretching works. "Rush" refers not just to my name but also to a key part of the technique, which requires that each stretch last for just two seconds. "Reverse" refers to my discovery that a sequence that *decreases* the intensity and range of movement *before* you stretch greatly improves your results. The Rush Reverse distills the key elements needed to induce muscle lengthening into a simple procedure that you can use anytime, anywhere, on its own, or in combination with other exercises. (See p. 38 for detailed instructions.)

As noted, most Western forms of exercise emphasize stressful movement of the muscles and the misguided "no pain, no gain" attitude. Safe stretching avoids harsh movements that trigger the production of large quantities of lactic acid in muscle fibers, which causes fatigue and tightness. Inhaling more oxygen lessens this fatigue, but it is not sufficient to counteract the negative effects of lactic acid. Rapid movement of the muscles also can cause excessive strain on the heart if it is already weak.

Thus, extreme muscle development is not necessarily a recipe for health. A healthy body requires balanced flexibility, stamina, strength, organ functioning, and mental control. In safe exercising, movements are gradual, often slow, always paired with their kinetic opposites, and coordinated with complementary breathing and relaxation. In safe stretching, you hold the stretch alertly for just two seconds, then release for a few seconds, then repeat the two-second stretch. Repetition adds a crucial aspect that gradually builds muscle strength and retrains your reflexes.

Stretching can benefit people of varying ages and in various physical conditions. Children, too, have fun doing exercises. Perhaps yours would like to practice along with you. Be sure to meditate on noncompetitiveness first, because children are usually much more flexible than adults.

Safe stretching is terrific for aging bodies. The most common early indication of physical aging is stiffening of the joints. Ease of movement is often assumed to be the province of the young. But stretching can counter- act this trend by careful attention to moving all the joints during exercise. Faulty alignment of the spine and poor balance can cause shortening of the ligaments and many other movement problems. Flexibility exercises help keep your spine in good alignment, and the low impact of controlled movements prevents strain to muscles and bones.

Several good reasons to do flexibility exercises are the mood and health benefits of increased oxygen and blood circulation. Slow

I feel sorry for someone who has to win at everything.
— Snoopy

movements combined with deep breathing achieve improved health better than fast, jerky ones. Efficient, coordinated movement develops as one practices safe stretching, because the balanced poses improve the central nervous system.

Women may have an easier time beginning than men because they are less apt to have practiced years of heavy bodybuilding sports, which shorten the tendons, flex primarily in a single direction, and leave a person muscle-bound. Also, women's hip joints are set farther apart than men's and can rotate in such a way that women can often assume complex positions with relative ease. This can be embarrassing to an otherwise athletic male.

Leave behind the idea of stable solutions. Built to last now means built to change.

— Stan Davis and
Christopher Meyer,
Blur

Of course, an overdeveloped sense of competition can spoil a workout for a student of either sex. Competition is not part of integrated flexibility training. Measure your progress only by your own sense of fulfillment.

As Deepak Chopra, MD, points out in his book *Ageless Body, Timeless Mind,* stress causes most of what we think of as signs of illness and aging. Exercise lowers your biological age and reduces stress so that your body can function well and look better at any age. Your degree of health and flexibility, not your age, determines how much you are able to do in life.

Use It or Fuse It

The way we stretch helps sculpt the shape of the muscles we develop and helps determine the quality of motion we display. You can move comfortably at any age if you move well each day. Physical flexibility requires proper movement of every joint in your body at least five days a week. If we do not move an area, a host of problems can occur: circulation gradually slows, waste materials build up rather than pass through, tendons and ligaments tighten and become brittle, skin loses its elasticity, muscle tone diminishes. The body's normal aging process includes loss of moisture content in the tissues. Our previously elastic muscle fibers clump together with connective tissue to cause stiffness. Unless we stretch, we dry up and fuse.

Ultimately, a joint can stiffen to the point of losing its ability to bend. Range of motion lessens, movements become jerkier, and comfort and pleasure in our body's locomotion wane. However, a simple cure for stiffness exists. Safe stretching separates the clumped cellular cross-links and encourages muscles to rebuild in healthy parallel structure.

Time to start stretching. Better yet, begin before you hurt in order to prevent such miseries. Anyone at any age can increase mobility. You simply need to follow the basic guidelines below and stay within your comfort zone to prevent strain.

Basic Guidelines

Begin exercising with slow, steady movement sequences that increase your heart rate and muscle range. To cool down, slow your range and pace. Take the following guidelines to heart so you won't have to take your muscles to the doctor.

- Do not hold an extreme stretch for longer than two seconds, or you will trigger shortening of the muscle.

> *Fast is fine, but accuracy is everything.*
> — Wyatt Earp

- Don't jerk, throw your limbs, or bounce; quick, rough moves tighten your muscles. Control your actions.

- Don't hold painful positions; this can tear your muscles.

- Don't exercise an injured area without consulting your physician.

- Don't favor one side or one direction of movement; this can lead to difficulties on the undeveloped side.

- Don't hold your breath; this starves your muscles of oxygen.

- Do move gently and smoothly; this builds strong muscles and burns fat more efficiently than movement at a fast pace.

- Bend gradually and stay warm to prevent strain.

- Pace yourself within your individual comfort zone.

- Notice where you tense muscles unnecessarily, such as shoulders, jaw, or hands, so that while exercising one muscle, you do not unconsciously stress another.

- Occasionally perform the routine with speed to increase aerobic effect and coordination.

- Sprinkle single short stretches and five-minute meditations throughout your day for relaxation breaks and stress management.

- Drink plenty of water. This increases your blood volume, thus circulation, thus relaxation.

- Experiment with stretching to music to keep your pace and to inspire you.

- Many stretching guides specify different routines for different sports. This is not necessary, because you need to limber your whole body to play any sport well.

- Do some exercises from all the sections, selecting your favorite exercises from each body area to make up your personal flexibility regimen.

- Generally, throughout exercises, breathe with your motion: inhale as you stretch out, exhale as you bend in or release.

- When exercising on your back, lie on the floor or on a firm pad for proper support.

MIND STRETCHING

Why Meditation?

The mind is like a muscle: use it or lose it. It is a body part and needs exercise to function well. Meditation is like a stretching exercise for the mind. When you start with meditation, everything that follows works better. The meditation process helps you empty your mind of surface thoughts so that deeper, more profound perspectives can float into consciousness. Meditation also allows us to relax and slow down our thoughts. The gaps between our thoughts gradually become longer and longer. It is during these gaps, free of judgment and emotion, that we find peace and clarity.

Nothing gives one person so much advantage over another as to remain always cool and unruffled under all circumstances.

— Thomas Jefferson

In Eastern development systems, conscious thoughts are considered to be mostly confused, dreamlike misinterpretations or subjective distortions of reality. We can learn to recognize spiritual truth, or reality, through the stages of meditation. In turn, yogis believe that truth shall make you free.

Every solid particle of matter is composed of 99.999 percent empty space.

— Deepak Chopra, MD,
Ageless Body, Timeless Mind

Stretching Your Pauses

Meditation is the exploration of the pauses between thoughts. The mind can find balance that is considered spiritually more real — that is, more divine — than thinking. This spiritual harmony beyond thought is described in the biblical phrase "the peace that passeth understanding."

If you can observe your thoughts as neither good nor bad, just there, and identify with the calm between your thoughts, your moods and perspectives will become more balanced. Practice a meditation method, such as Counting Breaths (see p. 87), for as long as you want. When you arrive at an alert, expansive peacefulness, remain in this space without using a meditation method. Resume the method only when you become distracted by thinking.

In advanced meditation, the student combines breathing and chanting with meditation in an attempt to move the physical spinal, or vital kundalini, energy up from the base of the spine to the top of the head. Partial movement of this kundalini energy produces only partial perception and stunted awareness. All the nerve centers must be awakened and unified to produce full spiritual understanding and action. This gradual process can take years, and the state of mental union can come and go. Someone who maintains a state of spiritual balance all the time is considered enlightened. Most of us see the light only briefly, but even small moments of clarity can illuminate a life.

See if you can develop the same nonjudgmental response to others that you are cultivating toward yourself during meditation. The choicest fruit of meditation is that your participation in the world becomes more peaceful and constructive.

Energy Flexing

Our energy systems need stretching along with our muscles and bones. Energy is a valued commodity. Even though we can't see energy, it doesn't occur to most of us to question whether energy is real, because we can feel it. Usually we have enough steam to perform our activities, but sometimes our power is not equal to our tasks. We'd like to be able to renew our energy at will, and we employ a variety of techniques in this effort. Asian disciplines can add valuable information to our Western endeavors because they offer detailed maps of the body's energy system.

> *Energy imbalance — its excess or insufficiency — is the root of illness.*
>
> — Yoshio Manaka, MD,
> *The Layman's Guide to Acupuncture*

In traditional Japanese medicine, philosophy, and martial arts, the term for energy is ki. Chinese medicinal and spiritual systems label energy chi. In Indian medical and spiritual terminology, the word for energy is prana, which is thought to come from the air we breathe.

In all cultures, energy level is one index of health. In Chinese medicine, appropriate energy flow through the body is considered the most important indicator and source of good health.

The Chinese medical system of acupuncture was developed more than four thousand years ago from observation that specific places on the body become sensitive or sore when a person is ailing. A map of these spots shows lines connecting the points that affect one another most directly. Westerners call these lines of energy pathways meridians. Western science acknowledges the existence of electromagnetic currents, or meridians, in the body that can affect health and can be measured by scientific equipment. The Chinese names for the negative and positive charges of electricity are yin and yang. Imbalance of these two currents in our bodies is seen as the root of all pathology.

Western doctors use electrostimulation treatments and physical therapy to revive damaged muscles. Asian medicine uses acupuncture stimulation and exercise. *The Layman's Guide to Acupuncture* is a helpful book for practical use.

> *Meditators have a biological age five to twelve years younger than their chronological age.*
> — Deepak Chopra, MD

Remember that as you exercise a body part, you stimulate the energy center located there. When you are stretching your muscles, you are balancing and recharging your whole electrical energy system. As you become comfortable with your stretching exercises, add awareness of the energy centers described in the following meditations as you perform the movements.

Chakra Meditation

The yoga chakra chart provides a clear, practical map of physical-emotional connections. Chakra is the name for a biological nerve center, or plexus. Understanding how our physical energy functions can improve our stretching process.

Each nerve center is thought to be a healing source for its biological function as well as related spiritual energy. An example is the heart chakra, located at the cardiac nerve center and allied to a person's sense of compassion. All centers need to be functioning well for the body and psyche to be in balance. Classic meditation calls for you to focus your attention on the energy center at the base of the spine and then to imagine stimulating each higher center and its associated functions as your attention rises to the top of the head. This is the natural sequence of energy movement.

1. ***Pelvic chakra.*** Base of spine and organs of elimination; center of basic health, survival, and rootedness. Pelvis and genital organs; center of sexual as well as artistic creativity.

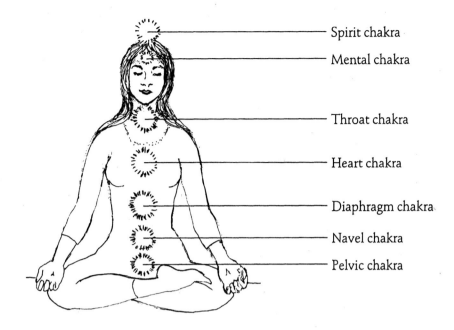

Spirit chakra

Mental chakra

Throat chakra

Heart chakra

Diaphragm chakra

Navel chakra

Pelvic chakra

2. **Navel chakra.** At belly button; center of body for balance and sense of self.

3. **Diaphragm chakra.** Digestive organs and belly area up to diaphragm; center of balance, identity, and outer-directed power.

4. **Heart chakra.** Cardiac plexus, thymus gland, and chest; center of love and compassion.

5. **Throat chakra.** Vagus nerve, thyroid gland, and cervical ganglion; center of communication.

6. **Mental chakra.** Pineal gland and "third eye" at center of forehead; center of mental perspective.

7. **Spirit chakra.** Top of head and pituitary gland; center of sense of connection with all creation.

Visualization

Visualization can be used as a form of practice that will improve your performance. Many Olympic and professional coaches add preworkout visualization of the athlete's body performing a perfect movement as part of cutting-edge training. Imagining something stimulates many of the same responses in your nerves and muscles as doing it. Visualize yourself doing an exercise or sport before the event. You can also use visualization throughout the day as a preventive technique by maintaining a healthy image of your body in top shape.

Imagine healthy, flexible images of your body to improve your physical condition and performance. The strength of your mind can revive flagging muscle power and help smooth tight muscles. If you have a torn ligament, allow yourself to see an image in your mind's eye of the current state of that body part, imagining what the area looks like fragmented and inflamed. Next visualize how it *should* be. Looking at anatomy charts is useful. Throughout the day bring this healthy picture of your ligaments and muscles to mind to encourage healing.

No one has yet calculated how many imaginary triumphs are silently celebrated by people each year to keep up their courage.

— Athenaeus, c. A.D. 200

The process of visualization is an ancient technique that various healers have used throughout history. Many medical doctors now use visualization training effectively to help cancer patients and injured athletes. Visualization is also useful for people who are in pain, too tired, or too sick to do other kinds of treatments or exercise.

Visualize Healing

Visualization can be used to explore an emotional or physical pain or a tight muscle. Imagine that you can shrink yourself and walk into your body to search and do internal maintenance. Don't preplan the story; try to simply let the events occur. They will.

Lie down, close your eyes, and relax your breathing. If you have a specific ache or pain you want to work on, locate it and then choose a natural body opening as your "entranceway." Imagine you can shrink yourself to about half an inch or smaller.

The journey in and out is just as important as the destination. Resist hurrying or missing any steps. You can talk out loud about what you are doing and how it feels to you. If you have a pain in your upper back you want to reach, you could enter through your mouth. Look around at the setting and describe it. "I am walking up to the mouth. I am crawling over the lips. As I let myself down inside, the surface becomes slippery. It's dark in here. I'm walking toward the back of the mouth on the teeth. They feel sharp and bumpy."

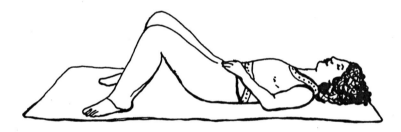

When you reach the back of the mouth, decide how to get down the throat and into the shoulder. "There's a deep hole here like a well. There's no way to get down except jump, but I don't know where I'll land." You can decide to go on or try another way. "I think I'll just jump." Describe your descent, what you see, how you feel. Almost always a surprise landing takes place; if not, pick something to catch on to to stop yourself when you feel you've fallen far enough.

When you land, decide how you're going to get to your sore muscle. You can swim through an artery or walk along a tendon. When you reach the sore muscle, look around. Describe what you see. Try to imagine a way you could massage the muscle by walking on it or squeezing it. Imagine you are doing this. Take your time.

When you have massaged to your satisfaction, begin your journey out of the body. Outside again, imagine you can expand to your normal size and merge with your larger body. Take a moment to check how the previously sore muscle feels now. Often it feels greatly relaxed.

MIND-BODY BASICS

The Way of Stretching assumes that each person's mind, body, and spirit need balanced attention in order to function fully. The Western definition of flexibility is the capacity to move muscles and joints through their complete range. The Eastern definition is a balance of physical and mental range. Modern scientific research on the interrelatedness of biological processes reflects this ancient wisdom. In *The Man Who Tasted Shapes,* Richard Cytowic, a Washington, D.C., medical doctor, sums up current computer research on the human brain: "Some experts in artificial intelligence now believe that without emotion, thinking is impossible."

> *It is not the strongest of the species that survive, nor the most intelligent, but the ones most responsive to change.*
> — Charles Darwin

Safe, integrated stretching is not meant to be a spectator sport. Your attention is inward. Each position is designed to awaken informative sensations in your body and to trigger a series of physical adjustments that improve your flexibility. More surprises come over time, as integrated techniques offer an endless process for refining your physical and mental capabilities.

Relaxation

Of the two types of muscles, voluntary muscles are those that can be moved at will and gain direct benefit during exercise. Involuntary muscles, however, cannot be moved at will and receive only referred benefit from exercise when you release a contraction of a voluntary muscle. Then, the involuntary muscle lengthens and returns to its starting position. You cannot act to force it to lengthen; you can only not contract. Relaxation is a state of physical inaction and mental release triggered by the absence of the brain's command to act.

You may have noticed that when you are physically active, your breathing is fast paced and moves muscles high in your chest. When you are quiet and focused, your breathing automatically slows down and sinks deeper in your body. If we intentionally change our breathing, we can induce a variety of mental states at will. In Eastern spiritual and physical development practices, the human mind is viewed as an unsteady element at the mercy of external influences. It requires calming and internal focus to function well.

Most of the energy for the body we get from the air we breathe, and not, as is commonly assumed, from food and water.

— Swami Vishnudevananda,
The Complete Illustrated Book of Yoga

We all know it's not easy to control our minds. Breathing techniques are effective brain regulators because we can program our nervous systems by altering our breathing. Breathing is one of the few automatic, unconscious body functions that also can be controlled consciously. This makes it an exceptional tool for mental development. Magdalene Proskauer — the San Francisco Jungian therapist who trained me in her analysis techniques — says, "The breath is a bridge to the unconscious."

Inhalation contracts your muscles slightly. Exhalation releases your muscles slightly. As you exhale, the diaphragm pushes up against the heart, slowing down the heart rate. Blood pressure decreases, as does stress on the rib cage, abdominal walls, and intercostal muscles. Relaxation ensues, and your tolerance for stretching is enhanced — as well as your sense of well-being.

Prana

Every complete exercise system includes some breathing exercises. Yoga offers a spectrum of breath patterns for different purposes. The variety of breathing exercises in this book is designed to improve awareness of the many parts of your breathing and to teach control over your cycles. The nostril breathing improves circulation and clears the mind. Some of the exercises tend to heat the body, and some to cool it. Prana Seals, or breath locks, complete and intensify the effects of the exercise.

As noted, prana is the Indian yoga name for the energy current or life force in our bodies that animates all living things. Breathing is the result of prana, or chi, movement. Our first and last breaths define our lifespan. When breathing stops altogether, it is evidence that the prana, or the vital force of the body, has departed.

Prana waves move in different patterns to permeate life at all levels, from rocks and plants to people and ideas. Thought is considered the finest and highest manifestation of prana's movement in human beings. The process of controlling vital energy through breathing is called *pranayama*. The purpose of learning this control is to encourage the mind to move to higher planes of thought and understanding.

Prana is equated with life energy or vitality; thus, the more prana we have circulating in our bodies, the healthier we are. The main storage area in the body for prana is the solar plexus nerve center, just below the navel. Exercises can train us to circulate the prana out to other parts of the body.

We take in vitality, or prana, from the air we breathe and store it in our bodies. Vital prana energy needs to move and to be evenly distributed throughout the body to produce health and balance. We can learn to control prana through conscientious practice of focused exercises. The laying on of hands is thought to be a transfer of prana current. Both physical and mental energy come from prana. All willpower and all healing arise from control of this energy. Yoga patterns for breathing are designed to help clear out your air passages, improve your control and discrimination, and bring more prana and oxygen through your body.

Breathing into Body Parts

We have modern technology that can locate and measure electromagnetic currents in the body. Centuries ago, yogis felt these subtle currents during their practice and included systems for directing the currents to deepen the energizing effects of their movements. You can do a simple exercise with your hands to feel these currents. The experience offers you a way to heighten the scope and extend the range of your movements and send energy all over your body. Initially, try this technique with your hands. Later you can try directing the energy to any part of your (or someone else's) body. Directing the breath is the key.

There are no miracles, only unknown laws.

— Saint Augustine

1. Sit comfortably, eyes closed, hands resting palms up on your knees. Relax any tense muscles you feel by imagining that each time you

exhale, a little more tension leaves your body. Allow your breathing to sink low in your body so that your belly puffs out a bit as you inhale and sinks back in as you exhale.

2. Now imagine what it would feel like if you could send your exhalation through the center of your body, through your torso, to massage your muscles from the inside. Allow your breath to bring warmth and air to any tight areas. As you breathe, oxygen is drawn into your body and spreads to various parts through your bloodstream.

3. As you exhale, imagine you can send air down through your shoulders and arms and eventually into your hands. What would it feel like if you could exhale down your arms and out the centers of your palms, through a spot about the size of a quarter?

4. Raise your palms so they are facing each other at about waist height. The increased circulation to your hands as a result of your breathing some-times brings a sense of warmth and tingling. The muscle relaxation and improved circulation allow the body's electric currents to move more easily. Can you feel any sense of this electric flow between your facing palms?

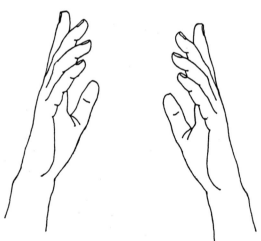

5. Some positions intensify the current flow. Allow your hands to move slowly in any direction they want. Try holding them different distances apart to see where the current feels stronger and where it weakens. You may sense a flexible shape to the air space. Sometimes it feels as though you were holding a ball between your hands.

6. The more you relax and direct your breathing down your arms, the stronger the sensation will become. You will notice that this process releases tension in your shoulders and arms. You can use this directed breathing to relax tight muscles in other parts of your body as well.

The quickest pain relief comes from doing the exercise while lying down, because you can give over the work of holding your weight to the bed or floor and concentrate your attention on relaxing. Adding a small movement to your breathing exercise can also increase its effectiveness at relieving pain. Synchronize the motions with your breathing. Inhale as you lift or stretch. Exhale as you release or bend. Most tension release occurs on the exhalation, as your muscles "let go."

Getting Started

Habits become entrenched after twenty-one days of repetition. Keep your new safe-stretching routine going for that long, and it will become an effortless part of your life. Start the day luxuriously by taking care of yourself first. Find a quiet place in your home with enough room to lie on a comfortable mat on the floor. The exercise area should be flat and smooth so you can move easily. Be sure you have enough privacy, so that you don't have to worry about being interrupted.

Begin your routine with a posture check. Simply stand and check your alignment and how your body feels. Are there any places where you feel stiff?

Then, starting with your feet, check the position of your body. Your feet should be facing forward and should be approximately as far apart as your shoulders.

Be sure you're not locking your knees. Bend your knees slightly to take some pressure off your calves and thighs.

Then check your abdomen and your pelvis to be sure that your stomach muscles are pulled in and your pelvis is *slightly* tilted forward.

Beginning at the base of your spine, move your awareness up your spine to see if it feels as though each vertebra is stacked comfortably on top of the others. In correct, fully erect posture, a line dropped from the ear should go through the outer tip of the shoulder, middle of the hip, back of the kneecap, and front of the ankle.

Cutting-edge techniques in Western flexibility training focus on reconditioning neurological mechanisms.
— Fernando Pagés Ruiz, *Yoga Journal*

When you come to the region of your upper back and chest, be sure that you're not bent forward and hunched into your chest. If you are, inhale and rotate your shoulders back to open up your chest, so that your upper back is not bent and your chest is not caved in. Be sure you're not leaning forward with your neck and that your chin is tucked under.

When you move you may notice that one side of your body will be looser and more relaxed than the other. See if that is consistent down the full length of your body. My right side is generally slightly tense and, therefore, less strong and not as flexible as my left.

As you move through the exercises, your circulation should pick up, and you should feel more awake. Starting slowly is important for good body tone, for preventing strains, and for an enjoyable exercise session. If you start with very vigorous exercise too quickly after you've been asleep or after a day of sedentary work, you'll be working against the condition of all of your muscles, which makes it more likely that you'll strain a muscle.

As you stand, try to imagine that a line is running from the center of the top of your skull through the center of your body down the length of your spine to the ground. This is the axis of all your movement. Imagine your limbs and muscles move around it as you exercise. You need to move the joints in your body or the synovial fluid will dry up, which causes your joints to become tense and tight. Moving them even a tiny bit each day will keep your joints producing this fluid, which keeps the joints flexible.

Beginning and Advanced

Beginning and advanced stretching do not necessitate different exercises. The difference lies in how you perform each stretch. When your muscles are cold, or if you are an exercise "beginner," move extremely slowly and stretch only a small amount. To make an exercise more "advanced," exercise for longer sessions and increase the frequency and range of your stretch, though never to the point of pain.

Stretch Your Pleasure

A study on stress conducted by Richard Lazarus and his colleagues at the University of California (UC), Berkeley, concluded that relatively minor yet frequent annoyances have a more destructive effect on our health than do grand-scale traumas. Perhaps this is because we don't pay attention to them. With stress, it's the little things that mean a lot.

> *What can we gain by sailing to the moon if we are not able to cross the abyss that separates us from ourselves?*
> — Thomas Merton

The study also found that small tension-relief sessions performed frequently throughout the day have the biggest effect on relieving stress. Make healing a way of life. Include short stretching and breathing breaks in each day's routine to keep the little molehills from becoming mountains. Take a moment to bend over in your chair and relax your back several times a day. Sprinkle brief stretches through-out your daily routine. They will add up to a big stress reduction.

> *Your mind, your feelings are in your body, and it's there, in your somatic experience, that feeling is healed.*
>
> — Dr. Candace Pert,
>   discoverer of the body's
>   opiate receptors

Another UC (Berkeley) study found that to be free of stress it's not enough to eliminate negative factors from your life. You have to *add* positive ones. This is a program worth lots of attention.

Fill your life with simple treats, luxuries, and happy experiences. Lavish your loved ones with frequent small signs of affection. Keep your body feeling great. Stretch your pleasure quota. Ease your mind and your muscles into it and begin.

Part II

Flexibility Exercises

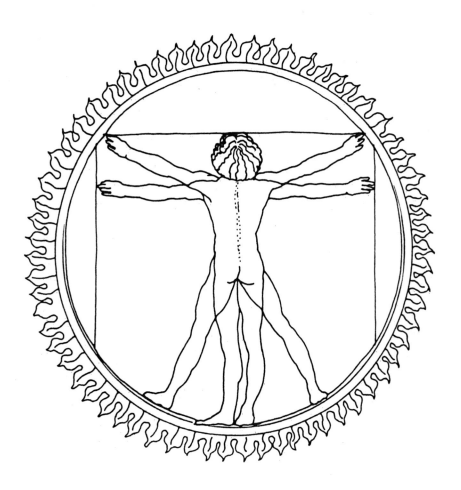

When you build a thing you cannot merely build that thing in isolation,
but must also repair the world around it, and within it, so that the larger world at
that one place becomes more coherent, and more whole;
and the thing you make takes place in the web of nature.

— Christopher Alexander, Sara Ishikawa, and
Murray Silverstein, *A Pattern Language*

ANATOMY OF A STRETCH

The human skeleton has 206 bones, all of which need exercise to maintain their mass. Without weight-bearing exercise to vibrate those bones correctly, they start to lose their density and become thinner and more fragile. Ligaments hold the bones together and are covered with cartilage. A joint's function is largely balance.

The body has six hundred different muscles, often paired in extenders and flexors. All these aspects of the body need exercise to function well.

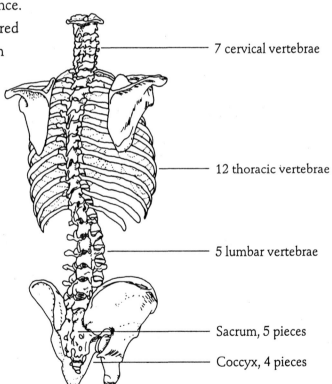

7 cervical vertebrae

12 thoracic vertebrae

5 lumbar vertebrae

Sacrum, 5 pieces

Coccyx, 4 pieces

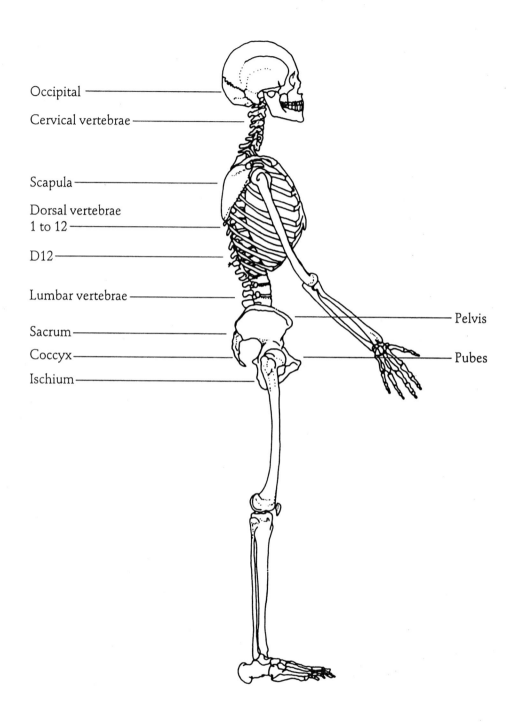

Occipital

Cervical vertebrae

Scapula

Dorsal vertebrae
1 to 12

D12

Lumbar vertebrae

Sacrum

Coccyx

Ischium

Pelvis

Pubes

Muscles are for movement. A muscle is an organ built from specialized tissues brought together to perform a function. Striated muscles are the kind that cause our bones to move and perform tasks. The smallest skeletal muscles are the tiny, barely visible ones in the middle ear. The largest skeletal muscle is the gluteus maximus, forming the buttocks.

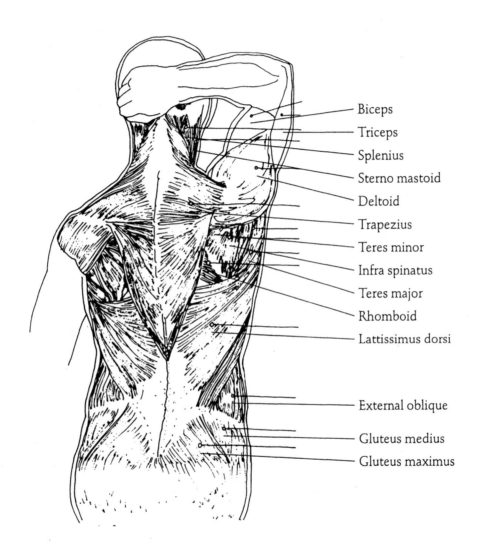

Biceps

Triceps

Splenius

Sterno mastoid

Deltoid

Trapezius

Teres minor

Infra spinatus

Teres major

Rhomboid

Lattissimus dorsi

External oblique

Gluteus medius

Gluteus maximus

Muscles have a buddy system and perform in pairs. One muscle group operates by contracting while its partner muscle group is relaxing. The ones that contract to move bones are called agonists. The opposing muscle groups that release and elongate to permit movement are called antagonists.

Muscles have a lot of nerve. Special sensors called muscle spindles run across the muscle fibers to notice how fast and far they elongate. The spindles fire nerve messages to trigger a contraction or stretch reflex if the movement threatens to tear the muscle. Other sensors, called Golgi tendon organs (GTOs), monitor muscles for possible injury. GTOs offer protection from tearing by signaling the complete release of the muscle. Some trainers try to strain an athlete's muscle to such an extreme that the GTOs sense overstimulation and signal a complete collapse of any holding in the muscle. This is one way to trigger muscle release and stretching. However, it is not recommended for use by anyone who is not specially and thoroughly trained. It is the emergency muscle release sought when a person is injured or in traction in the hospital. My preference for healthy muscle release is to seek a gentle muscle extension, triggered either by a relaxing exercise system or by the Rush Reverse sequence.

Connective tissue called muscle fascia groups muscle fibers together. The muscles' connective tissues are embedded in a gluelike matter called ground substance. Static stretching or inactivity, such as sitting in one position too long, can trigger the stretch reflex as well if the static state lasts long enough to cause discomfort. Hormones influence flexibility during life cycles. A hormone called relaxin, which loosens the ligaments of the lower back and hips, is released in a pregnant woman's body.

Water levels and body chemicals can affect flexibility. Dehydration and restriction of ground substance increase as we age and limit our flexibility. We can regain this flexibility, however, with stretching.

Muscle Myths and Facts

Myth: In order to improve a muscle's flexibility, I must increase the muscle fiber's elasticity.

Fact: Almost everyone's muscle fibers already have enough elastic range to perform even the most extreme position. Tight, short muscles are mainly a mental limitation. Your brain controls the lengthening of your muscles. To best improve flexibility, you need to learn to release the nerve mechanism that relaxes a tight muscle.

Myth: In order to improve the flexibility of my joints, I should stretch my tendons (which connect bone to muscle) and ligaments (which bind bone to bone inside the joint capsule).

Fact: Tendons and ligaments have almost no tolerance for stretching (4 percent) before they tear. Stretching muscle fascia, however, improves mobility. Muscle fascia, the connective tissue that separates and groups muscles into working units, is the most crucial tissue to stretch and also the only flexibility-limiting component that you can stretch safely.

Myth: If I extend a muscle beyond its current range and hold the stretch position, I'll increase its range.

Fact: Muscles that are overextended don't lengthen; they shorten. After just three seconds of stretching, an involuntary reflex — the "stretch reflex," or myostatic reflex — is triggered. This reflex pulls your muscle back to protect it from tearing. *The only way to safely increase a muscle's range is to relax it and then extend it for repeated two-second intervals.* Only gradual movement allows full range of motion, prevents strain, and builds stamina. This all-around flexibility is important because tightness in one area can cause problems and imbalances in another area.

Myth: If I stretch my muscles into a new position once today, tomorrow I'll be able to equal or exceed that position.

Fact: Doing an exercise once does not change your range. Repeating it several times in a row does. Moving in and out of the same posture several times triggers neurological retraining of your muscles. Ideally, the exercise should include some contraction element because, according to Gary Kraftsow, founder of the American Viniyoga Institute, "alternating between contracting and stretching is what changes the muscle." It's important to use the contraction and release to develop strength.

Myth: I should inhale as I stretch.

Fact: When you inhale, your muscles tighten slightly, which would reduce a stretch slightly. Exhaling releases tension, thus helping to lengthen a stretch.

Myth: Stretching is good for you.

Fact: What most of us have done as "stretching" (pushing a muscle beyond its range) is bad for us. To be safe, we should substitute "lengthening." Do this by gentle relaxation of the muscle, followed by two-second extension of range. See the Rush Reverse, below, for details.

The Rush Reverse

I invented the Rush Reverse system in order to facilitate training the body to stretch by relaxing rather than by straining. The Rush Reverse offers a simple way to incorporate healthy muscle-range increase into your existing activities. It does not require that you learn a whole new set of exercises. Reverse stretching can be applied to any movement, small and simple or long and complex.

Perform a reverse stretch, a sequence of minimizing and reversing range of movement, *before* you try to increase your range of motion. Choose whichever motion you want to improve and *decrease* the intensity and speed, performing it three times, doing less by half each time until you can barely feel you are moving. And last, perform your first motion to check whether your range has increased.

Include Breathing into Body Parts (see p. 22) with the Rush Reverse method to increase focus. Exhale at the moment of your actual stretch. In general, as you move, exhale any time you fold forward, and inhale as you open up or lean back. This is natural because the lungs get smaller as they expel air and puff up as they take in air. For long movement sequences, perform the exercise very slowly, smoothly, and always below your pain threshold. As when balancing a bowl of water while walking, you are continually threatening to spill over into strain, but you constantly right the balance by tiny adjustments that maintain ease. Whenever you feel a spot in your movement that is too tight, perform the Rush Reverse for that specific portion, then resume your normal sequence. This gentle approach to exercise enables you to "trick" your muscles into lengthening by making the stretching so small and so brief that no cramping is triggered. You will increase your range of motion without pushing as the nerves signal the muscle to relax more and more.

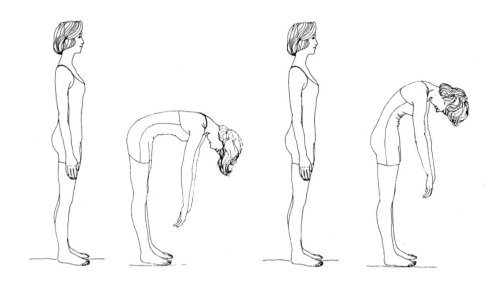

The Rush Reverse:

1. Perform a simple movement, such as leaning over while standing and trying to touch your toes. First, as you exhale, lean over toward your toes as much as you comfortably can. Notice how far past your knees your hands go. Crucial: hold the extreme range of the stretch for only two seconds. Then release the motion as you inhale, and relax back to standing. A two-second stretch may sound short, but since a nerve impulse takes just one hundred-thousandth of a second to cross a synapse, two seconds is plenty of time to send the message for the muscle to lengthen — and it's a second too short to trigger cramping.

2. Perform the same motion, but lean over only half as far as your first stretch. Relax back to standing as you exhale.

3. Perform the same motion a third time, but only half as far as the second time, or barely at all. Relax back to standing.

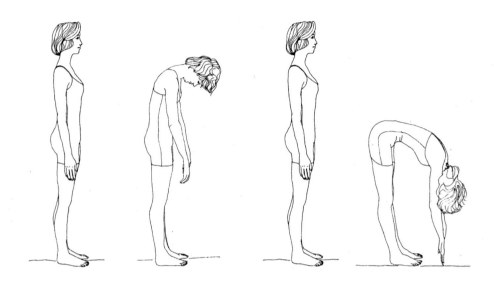

4. Now repeat step one by leaning forward as far as you comfortably can and trying to touch your toes. Your range should have increased noticeably. Without stressing or tightening, by gently performing the stretch in reverse, you will relax and lengthen your muscles and tendons, allowing a greater range of movement without strain or cramping.

Key Exercises and Body Treats

The first four exercises for each body area are tagged with a small key design (🗝). If you have limited stretching time, do the first four moves of each of the seven chakra areas to form a short limbering routine that encompasses your whole body's key stretch areas. Specific sports stretching routines can be built easily: do the first four key exercises of a body-area section and then perform typical motions from your selected sport (for instance, a golf swing or a soccer kick) in the Rush Reverse to lengthen your range in challenging positions.

After you have tried all the exercises in a chapter, select your favorites. The movements are mostly simple and familiar so that you can choose whether you prefer to perform them in the Rush Reverse sequence or in your regular manner. Any way you do them, include the Breathing into Body Parts process to enhance your limbering and your focus.

The exercises in this part of the book are organized in the yoga chakra framework of grouping functional areas and their related emotions and promoting balance of opposing muscle groups. Yoga is the most time-tested, versatile, and complete of all the sophisticated, gentle body-development systems. It also offers the clearest map of the mental aspect of exercise by including meditation, breathing, and nervous system (or chakra) balancing.

The meditations focus on the psychological associations of each body area to clear any related mental tensions connected to the physical ones.

Don't forget to visualize yourself performing an exercise before you do it. This is a form of practice and will improve your ability.

Aromatherapy can be a soothing addition to your body program. The pure essential oils extracted from plants can be mixed into pure body oils, such as almond, to create your own massage oils. Held in infusers or simply in small glass bowls, they impart their delicate scents to improve the ambience of your workout space. Be sure to use only pure, natural essential oils for aromatherapy. Breathing synthetics does not give your body the benefits of the real plant oil and might cause discomfort. Essential oils are concentrated, intensely fragrant, and relatively inexpensive, especially when you consider how they are made. One ton of citrus blossoms is required to produce two pounds of essential oil. Certain scents can help heal specific medical conditions. The scents listed with the exercises are all hypoallergenic and matched to the healing needs of each indicated body area. Enjoy!

FIRST CHAKRA STRETCH AREA
Feet, Legs, Lower Back

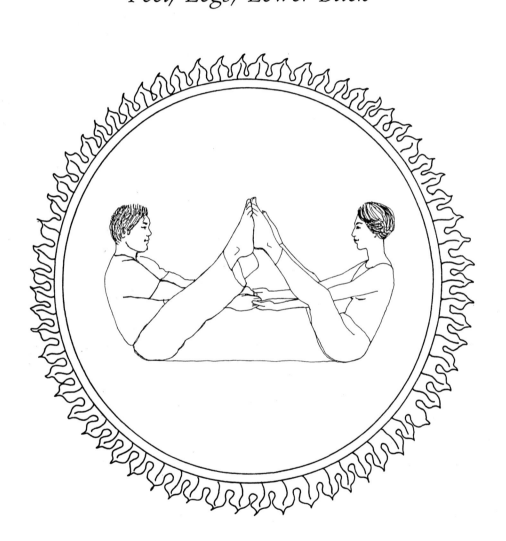

The first chakra, or energy center, is focused in the lower back and also includes the legs, feet, and organs of elimination. To stand upright, humans balance on three points on the foot that touch the ground: the heel and the outer and inner edges of the ball of the foot. Five pairs of lumbar nerves control your legs and feet. The nerves in your lower back spread into the abdomen and pelvis as well as down the legs, so limbering these areas improves digestive functions as well as movement of the back and legs.

Mind-Body Connection

If you understand the psychological connections of a body part, you can increase flexibility exercises for the area to relax emotional as well as physical tension. You can also explore these connections as you meditate.

Physiologically, feet are an extremely intense zone because nerves from all over the body culminate there. Thus, foot flexibility can relax nerves and send renewed energy to all parts of your body. Structurally, feet are essential to the support of your body when you are standing. Feet are, therefore, associated with our ability to be physically, as well as spiritually, "upright." When you feel like running away but have to stand your ground, a foot exercise can help bolster your resolve and courage.

Just as a strong foot represents a solid stand in the face of life's adversities, an injured foot represents a chink in our powers. The leg helps a person stand erect and, thus, is a symbol of being firm, of supporting, founding, and raising to new heights.

Psychologically, the feet represent our relationship to the earth. The feet affect how secure we feel about life's basic necessities, home, family, and social order. The organs of elimination cleanse the body of excess at the most basic level and are, thus, associated with this chakra and with life's most essential functions and routines.

First Chakra Meditation

Sit comfortably cross-legged on a mat on the floor. Place a small pillow or rolled towel under your tailbone to tilt you forward so that you can sit easily upright without tensing your lower back muscles.

I prayed for 20 years but received no answer until I prayed with my legs.
— Frederick Douglass

Silently ask yourself a series of questions that you think will increase your awareness of your sense of security and how to nourish it. Allow all the answers to surface and then fade until no more answers come. Then move on to the next question.

First Chakra Stretch Tips

- Breathe normally as you move. Do not hold your breath.

- Bend your knees slightly when standing.

- Do not bounce while stretching. This tightens your muscles.

- Slow and moderate-speed workouts burn more fat than fast ones.

- Stretch your tighter side first and longest.

- Align your knee directly over your foot as much as possible, especially when bending your leg.

- Keep your toes in line with the angle of the whole leg; do not point your toes in or out from the leg line.

- Our bodies have to be well hydrated before exercise for the muscles to be able to move in their full range of motion. Be sure to drink enough water or juice every day or to eat hydrated foods such as fruits.

- Remember the Rush Reverse (see p. 36): reverse stretching can help you increase your flexibility and range of motion, and it can be applied to any movement, small and simple or long and complex.

Aromatherapy

Aromatherapy essential oils that help heal disorders of the first chakra area include lavender vera, East Indian sandalwood, patchouli, Canadian balsam, jasmine, rosewood, and damask rose. Using lavender vera as an aromatherapy scent is a well-established folk remedy for shock, vertigo, and depression. The oil also helps cure athlete's foot, insect bites, and muscular aches such as lumbago.

First Chakra Stretches

TWINKLE TOES

These motions loosen the muscles in your feet, ankles, and knees.

1. Stand on your left foot, keeping your right heel on the ground. Point the toes of your right foot toward your left foot. Then pivot on your right heel so that the toes of your right foot point to the right. Repeat this motion several times with one foot. Switch and stand on your right leg and make the motion with your left foot.

2. This next movement is also done with your weight on one leg. Place the toe of your left foot on the ground so that the left heel is raised. Point your left heel toward your right toe. Now pivot on the ball of your left foot so that your left heel is pointing out away from your body and your left knee comes in toward your right knee. Repeat for the other side.

3. Stand with your weight on your left leg. Keeping the heel of your right foot on the ground, lift the ball of the foot up and fan your toes out as far as they will stretch. Then wiggle and bend them. Do this with your other foot.

4. Now lift one foot at a time off the floor and make circles with your ankles.

⚷ LEG LEANS

This movement focuses on stretching inner thigh muscles and the Achilles tendon, in your heel. To protect your knees from strain, be careful not to extend your knee beyond your foot.

Left

1. Standing up, place your hands on your hips. Face forward and inhale. Shift your weight onto your right leg, exhale, and bend the right knee. Stretch your left leg out to your left. Flex the left toes up, and bend the right knee more to accentuate the leg muscle stretch. Try to keep your torso upright; resist the impulse to lean forward.

2. Inhale as you roll your weight onto your left foot. Lean your body a bit to your left to center your weight on both feet again. You should be standing in the center as you began, with neither leg stretched to the side.

Right

3. Now lean farther to your left as you bend that knee and exhale.

4. Stretch your right leg out to your right. Flex the toes up.

5. Inhale as you return to your center stance.

Begin the whole sequence again to your right, but this time do not stop in the center between leans. Alternate right and left in one smooth, continuous motion.

SIDE LEG LIFT

1. Lying down, roll onto your side; align your spine and your body so that you're not arched at the waist or along your back. Rest your head on your lower extended arm. Place the palm of your upper arm in front of your chest for balance.

2. Inhale and lift both legs off the floor a comfortable few inches.

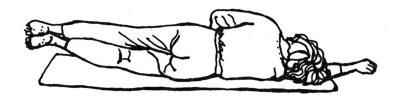

3. Then raise your upper leg as high as you can. Be sure that when you lift your legs you don't bring them forward and that you're keeping your body in a straight line.

4. Brings the legs together and then lower both.

5. Roll over and do the same exercise on the other side.

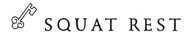 # SQUAT REST

This position opens hip joints to release pressure on the lower back as you lengthen the hip, leg, and back muscles. It relieves pinching of the sciatic nerves leading from the base of the spine, across the hips, and down the legs.

1. Standing with your feet shoulder width apart, bend your knees and squat. Try to keep your heels flat on the floor and parallel rather than turned out.

2. Press your elbows or forearms outward on the insides of your knees so your hip joints are stretched a bit. As you rest, your forehead can lean forward onto your clasped hands.

3. Gradually relax so that the position, rather than muscle tension, is holding you in place.

4. Stand up slowly, raising your shoulders and head last.

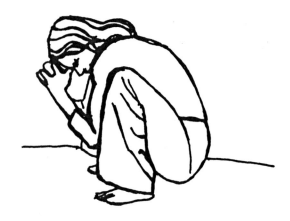

LEG LIFT STANDING

This movement helps loosen back muscles and hamstrings. Stand erect. Inhale as you raise one knee gently and pull it toward your chest with your hands. Exhale as you release your grip and let your knee move away from your chest, and slowly lower your leg to the floor again. Repeat with your other leg.

A limbering variation is to raise your knee and, as you exhale, lower your leg straight out in front of you, toes up and heels pressed out. Do several forward leg extensions as you exhale. Inhale between lifts as you bend your knee. Then relax your leg and foot. Try making these leg lifts to the side and to your rear several times. Keep your standing balance by staring at one spot in front of you at eye level as you lift.

Corrective Rests

If, while doing your exercises, you feel any pain or stress, stop immediately, take several deep breaths, and curl up into a fetal position on your side on the floor, which is the least stressful position for your back.

Or, if it feels comfortable, squat and curl in with your arms between your knees, clasping your hands and resting your forehead on them. Then rock back and forth (not side to side) in this position as you breathe.

An excellent lower-back release is to lie on the floor with the weight of your lower legs (from the knees down) on a bench or chair.

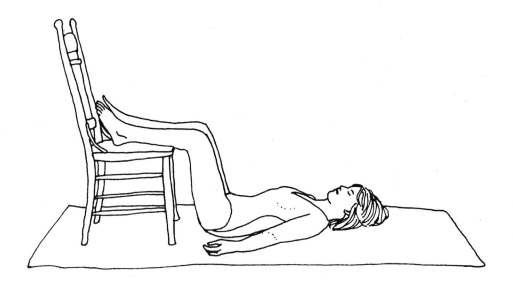

FLAPPER KNEES

This motion helps keep your knee and thigh muscles flexible.

1. Standing, place your feet about shoulder width apart. Press both knees outward to the sides, away from each other.

2. Keeping your feet stationary, draw both knees in until they touch.

3. Press both knees outward again. Alternate directions several times.

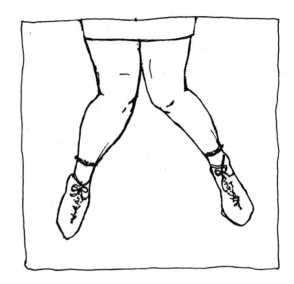

HEAD TO KNEES

With this exercise your back and leg muscles will become more limber, so that eventually you will be able to touch your head to your knees and hold your toes with your fingers. It may seem impossible at first, but gradually it will become easier. Each time, stretch only as far as is comfortable so you do not strain your leg muscles. Keep your knees slightly bent to avoid back strain.

1. Sit on the floor with your legs extended in front of you. Exhale as you bend at the waist and lean forward over your legs. Reach for your toes. Rest here a while and breathe normally.

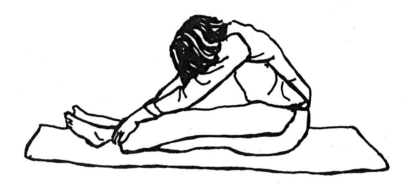

2. Inhale as you raise your arms above you and straighten your spine. Breathe through your nose. Relax your arms at your sides.

COBRA

This movement lengthens and strengthens the abdomen and back muscles, particularly those of the lower back. Use this stretch after forward extensions, such as Head to Knees, to balance the muscle movements.

1. Lie flat, face to the floor, and rest your forehead on your hands in front of you. Bend your elbows and slide your hands, palms down, to either side of your shoulders. Keep your feet together and your elbows close to your sides.

2. Inhale through your nose as you roll your head and neck back and up so you can look toward the ceiling. Keep your shoulders low and relaxed as you begin to raise your chest off the floor. Try to use your arms as little as possible so the muscles working are mainly in your back and abdomen.

3. Arch your spine backward as far as is comfortable while keeping your abdomen on the floor as much as possible. Hold this position a while.

4. Reverse the process as you unroll until you are lying down again, exhaling.

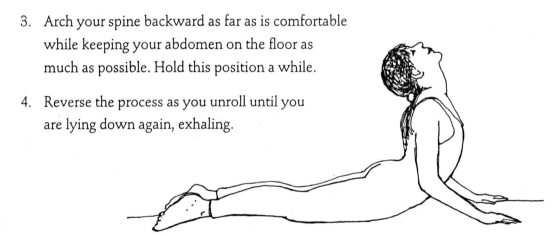

GROIN GROUNDING

This posture can help relax the hip joints and groin muscles. It also loosens the knees and thighs. Do not press your joints beyond a comfortable stretch or you can strain the muscles and ligaments.

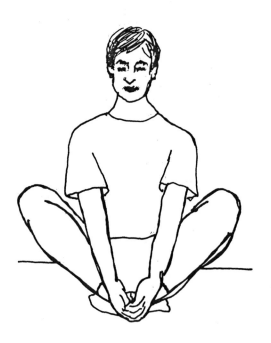

1. Sit comfortably on the floor with your knees bent and your legs crossed at the ankles. Then uncross your ankles and place the soles of your feet together; hold your toes with clasped hands. Use the grasp of your feet to help you keep your spine straight.

2. Exhale as you lightly press your knees out and down toward the floor. Inhale as you draw them up toward the ceiling. Move slowly and comfortably, without bouncing.

THIGH FLEX

1. Sit comfortably on the floor with your legs crossed loosely and your palms resting on your knees.

2. Place a firm, slim pillow or mat under your tailbone. This will afford your torso the slight lift forward that it needs to straighten rather than curve backward.

3. When you have found the proper lift, you can sit without holding up with your back or leg muscles. The alignment of the vertebral column will support you without muscle effort, and you can relax more deeply. Tilt your knees down toward floor, then release.

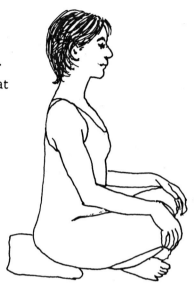

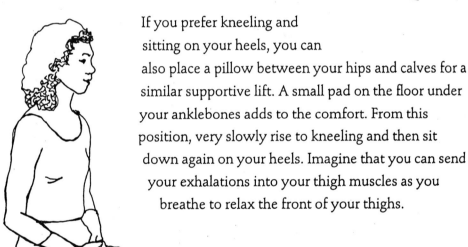

If you prefer kneeling and sitting on your heels, you can also place a pillow between your hips and calves for a similar supportive lift. A small pad on the floor under your anklebones adds to the comfort. From this position, very slowly rise to kneeling and then sit down again on your heels. Imagine that you can send your exhalations into your thigh muscles as you breathe to relax the front of your thighs.

FULL REST

It should be so simple to lie down and relax. However, sometimes we're too tense to fully release all our muscles. If so, the following gentle sequence should do the trick. It can also help you sleep more deeply.

1. Lie on your back on a flat surface with your arms resting at your sides. Your palms can be up or down, whichever relaxes your shoulders more. Try to clear your mind of thoughts and focus on the feelings in your body. Make a mental note of how your body feels lying on the floor. Starting with your feet, notice which parts of your body touch the floor and which parts arch away. Do you feel tilted in any direction?

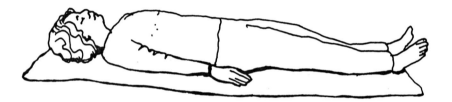

2. Flex and release each joint and muscle, working up from your feet to your head. Inhale as you flex; exhale as you release. Allow your breathing to massage you from the inside, as though you could exhale through your body and into any tight areas to soften them.

3. If you are still awake when you reach your head, compare how your body feels now to when you started.

PYRAMID FOR TWO

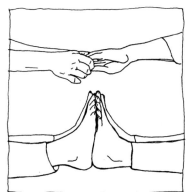

1. Sit facing each other with your legs relaxed in front of you on the floor. Inch your hips forward so that you can join hands, press the soles of your feet together, straighten your backs, and look steadily into each other's eyes. Slide your hips forward as you bend your knees more.

2. Gradually straighten your legs and raise your feet higher, above your clasped hands. Keep a firm hand grip for balance. Inhale and exhale deeply several times as you secure your pose. Maintain your gaze, blinking as little as possible.

3. Before lowering your legs as you exhale, inhale deeply once and hold your breath to a count of sixteen.

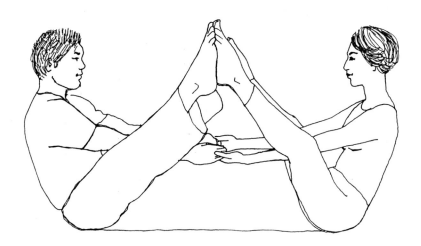

SECOND CHAKRA STRETCH AREA
Hips, Buttocks, Abdominals

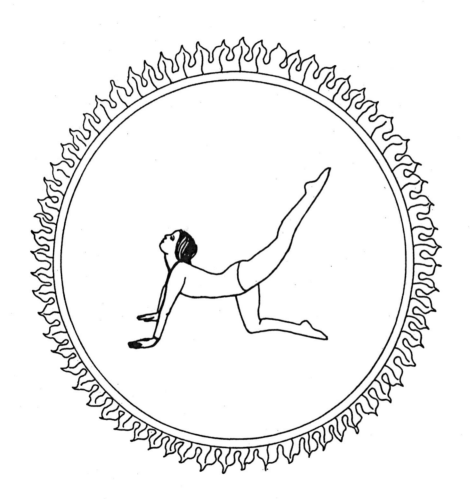

The energy center of the second chakra is in the lower back, hips, buttocks, and lower abdominals. The back has more than eighty muscles, divided into three main groups, that help secure the spine and offer a wide range of bodily motion. The spine is a stack of thirty-three vertebrae that curve in three places and form a protective case for the spinal cord, the body's major nerve pathway. Six pairs of nerves from the sacrum and coccyx control your pelvic organs and buttocks muscles. The sexual organs rest inside the lower abdomen, protected by the bones of the pelvis and lower back and by the muscles of the abdomen.

Lovemaking burns about 210 calories.

Mind-Body Connection

If you understand the psychological connections of a body part, you can increase flexibility exercises for the area to relax emotional as well as physical tension. You can also explore these connections as you meditate. The psychological association of the second chakra is a relationship to sex and all kinds of creativity.

Second Chakra Meditation

Sit comfortably on a mat on the floor with your knees bent and legs crossed. Place a small pillow or rolled towel under your tailbone to support your spine and tilt your weight slightly forward. This angle should allow you to balance and sit up straight without having to tense your back muscles. The head, neck, and torso are in a straight line, while the lower back is slightly arched.

I see all gods within your body.
— Bhagavad Gita

Rest your hands, palms up, on your knees. Touch your thumb to the forefinger to form a loose circle. Close your eyes. Relax your breathing so that you can feel movement low in the muscles of your abdomen as you puff out (inhale) and sink in (exhale). If you can do so comfortably, reposition your legs into a full lotus (knees bent, ankles crossed on top of each other). Otherwise, remain in a loose lotus. Visualize that your pelvic area and abdominals are warmed by a rose-gold light from within.

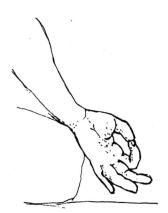

Second Chakra Stretch Tips

- Breathe normally as you move. Do not hold your breath.

- Tighten your buttocks muscles while performing back exercises to help protect your lower back.

- Tighten and pull in your abdominal muscles before performing stomach and back exercises.

- Relax your arms, hands, and shoulders while exercising your stomach.

- Remember the Rush Reverse (see p. 36): reverse stretching can help you increase your flexibility and range of motion, and it can be applied to any movement, small and simple or long and complex.

Aromatherapy

Aromatherapy essential oils that help heal disorders of the second chakra area include orange blossom, East Indian sandalwood, cardamom, lavender vera, marigold, and vetiver. Vetiver is known in Sri Lanka and India as "the oil of tranquility." The scent is healing and is used in incense, massage oils, and bath oils to relax nervous tension and muscular aches and to relieve depression and stress. It soothes sprains, stiffness, and muscle pains.

Second Chakra Stretches

HIP FOLDS

Use this exercise to limber the muscles of your hips, waist, and lower back.

1. While lying on your back, bring your arms up behind your head, with your palms under your head and your elbows out. Keep the small of your back on the floor and your stomach pulled in. Inhale and bend your knees.

2. Exhale and roll your knees and hips to your right. Now inhale as you bring both your knees up to the center again. Exhale and roll your knees and hips to the left. Inhale as you come to the center. Repeat this cycle slowly several times to limber the muscles on the sides of your hips.

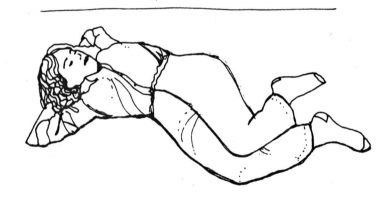

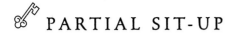 PARTIAL SIT-UP

This exercise strengthens your abdominal muscles, which are a major support for your lower back. It also strengthens your lower back muscles.

Lie on the floor, knees bent, feet flat. Keep your stomach muscles pulled in and the small of your back pressed down during this exercise. Resting your palms on your chest, inhale as you raise your head, neck, and upper back off the floor. Press your shoulders down, away from your ears. Push into the floor with your feet. With elbows slightly bent outward, extend your palms toward your knees. Hold your arms outstretched parallel with the floor as you count to two. Next reach about an inch forward with your arms. Count to two. Release the stretch by leaning back a few inches. Breathe. Then, on an exhalation, stretch forward again for two seconds. Do sequences for as long as is comfortable. Then very slowly return to the supine position by lowering your back, then your neck, then your head, and finally your arms to the floor.

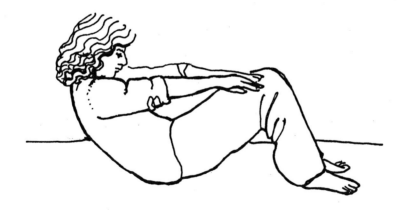

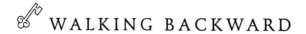 # WALKING BACKWARD

Another exercise for limbering and strengthening your hip, buttocks, and lower back muscles is done lying on your stomach.

1. Fold your hands under your chin and rest your head on them, or wedge your palms under your hip bones, whichever position is more comfortable for your lower back.

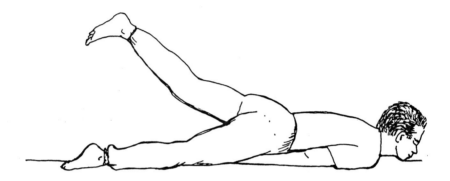

2. As you inhale, raise one leg behind you, keeping the leg straight. Do not arch your back as you lift. Lower and hold the leg about twelve inches from the floor for a count of two.

3. Then lower your leg to the ground slowly as you exhale.

4. Repeat with the other leg.

PELVIS ARCH

This exercise helps to strengthen and limber the gluteus maximus muscles in your buttocks, which help support your spine. It can also help prevent swayback, or lumbar spinal curve.

1. Lie flat on your back with your arms relaxed at your sides. Bend your knees and, keeping your feet flat on the floor, slide your heels toward your hips. Flatten your entire spine against the floor. Raise your buttocks and then your back off the floor by contracting the muscles of your abdomen and buttocks. Inhale as you lift.

2. Exhale as you lower your pelvis again. Lower the vertebrae at your upper back, then your waist, and then the rest down to your tailbone. Work up to the full tilt gradually.

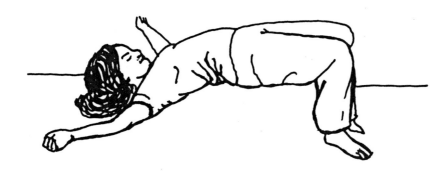

KNEE KISS

Any version of this pose gives a good stretch to the whole spine. Do as much as you can without pain today, and tomorrow your range will be greater.

1. Lie flat on your back. Exhale as you bend one leg and pull it toward your chest while keeping the other leg straight on the floor.

2. Simultaneously curve your neck and upper back and draw your forehead toward your bent knee. Rest in this position for a few breaths.

3. Lower your head and leg slowly as you exhale. Repeat the sequence with the other leg.

Try lifting both legs at the same time for a double stretch.

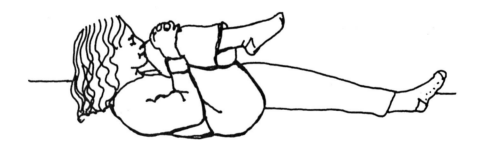

INCHWORM

This exercise lengthens your hip, buttocks, and leg muscles.

1. Begin on your hands and knees and raise yourself onto your palms and feet so that your back is arched.

2. Keeping your knees straight and your belly drawn in, walk your hands forward without letting your hips sag.

3. Keeping your legs straight, walk your feet with baby steps toward your hands, going as far as you can without bending your knees.

4. Repeat this cycle of the inchworm walk until you have covered several yards.

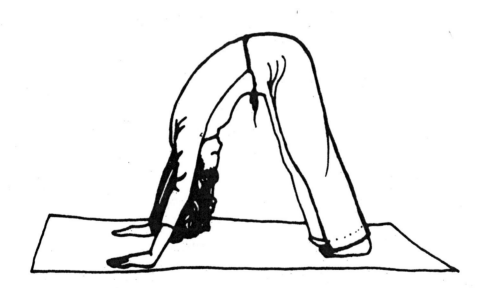

SQUAT REST

The next position is good for your whole body. In rural America it's often referred to as the Arkansas squat. In many countries where it is not customary to use chairs, this is the position people sit in all the time. It keeps your hip and knee muscles particularly flexible. Sitting on chairs tends to allow the hip muscles to atrophy. This exercise also helps relax your back and your hip joints.

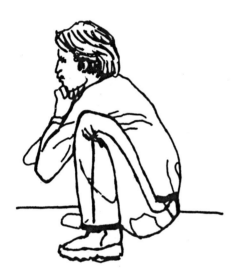

1. Standing with your feet flat on the floor, bend your knees and squat down so that your derriere is almost touching the floor. Lean your torso forward. Position your shoulders between your knees and clasp your hands.

2. Rest with your chin on your hands in this position. You can also take your thumbs, place them on either side of the bridge of your nose near your eye sockets, and rest your forehead forward on your thumbs. If it's comfortable for you, this position can be useful for meditation.

HIP DANCE CIRCLES

While standing with your hands on your hips,
rotate your pelvis laterally in full circles in
one direction and then another. Keep
your belly flat. Breathe in sync with your
movement. Gently increase your range
of motion to relax your thighs, hips,
and abdomen and smooth out the
circles as you include more body
parts in the rotation.

HIP TURNS

Right

This stretches your hip and waist muscles.

1. Stand with your feet about shoulder width apart. Place your hands on your hips and look to your right.

2. Shift your weight onto your left leg with the knee slightly bent so you can tilt your right hip up a bit toward your shoulder. Bend to your right at the waist and drop your right shoulder toward your right hip.

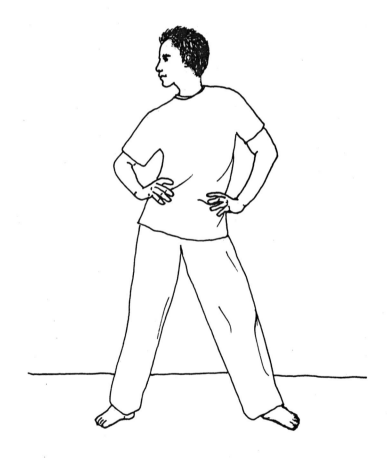

Middle

This movement stretches your waist, abdomen, and hip muscles.

3. Tuck your fanny under and press your pelvis forward.

4. Roll your hips from the right toward the rear until your fanny is pressed out behind you.

Left

This action relaxes your hip joints, knees, and shoulders.

5. Roll your hips to your left. Look to your left. Drop your left shoulder. Tilt your left hip up as you bend at the waist and your weight shifts to your right leg.

6. Complete the circle by rolling your hips to the center again. Face forward.

Do several full Hip Turns in a row with no break in between. Try to keep the movement smooth and continuous.

Around Again

Make a full Hip Turn sequence in the opposite direction. Start by rolling your hips to your left, then back, then right, then to the middle and front.

HALF LOTUS

This pose helps release your pelvic muscles and flexes your leg joints.

1. Sit on the floor with one leg extended, the other with the knee bent.

2. Place the foot of the bent leg up on the opposite thigh as close to the hip joint as is comfortable.

3. Fold the other leg under the upper thigh of the bent leg. Rest here and breathe.

4. Repeat with the other leg.

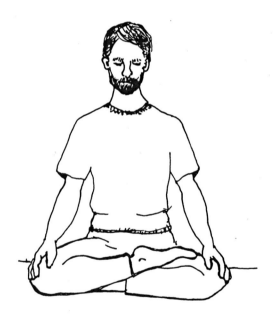

Relaxation

Between exercises, lie on your back on the floor with your knees bent and relax completely as often as needed. Do this also throughout your exercising so that you never strain yourself, you always keep within your limits, and you are refreshed rather than exhausted by what you're doing.

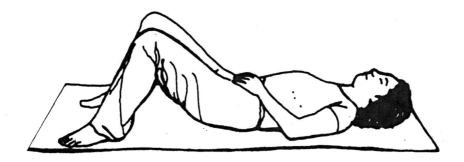

After you finish your exercises, lie on your back, knees bent, feet on the floor. Or try raising your knees over your chest, palms slipped between your calves and thigh muscles, holding your knees comfortably. Close your eyes. Let your breathing relax your torso and your stomach; relax all the muscles in your body and experience the pleasure and benefit of the exercises you've done. Feel your whole body tingling slightly and feel the increased suppleness of your muscles.

THIRD CHAKRA STRETCH AREA
Abdominals, Rib Cage, Diaphragm

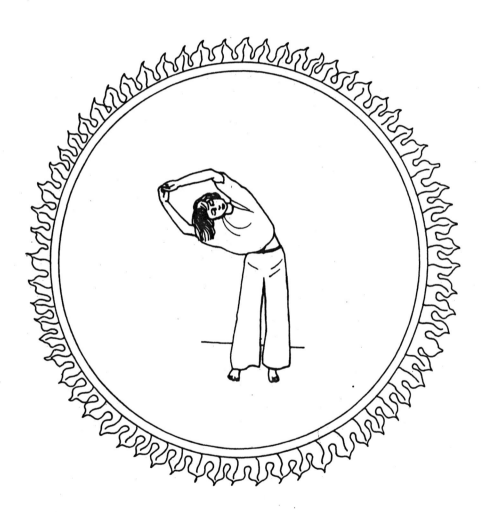

The third chakra is centered in the upper abdominal and diaphragm regions. Twelve spinal vertebrae just below the neck extend around the torso of the body to form the rib cage that protects the lungs, heart, and upper abdominal area.

Mind-Body Connection

If you understand the psychological connections of a body part, you can increase flexibility exercises for the area to relax emotional as well as physical tension. You can also explore these connections as you meditate.

The belly is the place of digestion and, thus, is a symbol of transformation, of bringing exterior material inside to change it into nourishment, "food for the soul." The round belly with the navel at its center can be seen as a symbol of the concentric circles of heaven and earth, with a dot at the ultimate center representing God, or the Creator. Psychologically, the belly represents the center of our bodies, the location of inner and outer balance and our sense of individual solidity. Meditating on your navel represents bringing your focus to the point of unity with the Divine.

The diaphragm is the spot in the center of our chest to which most of us point when we want to indicate "me." Psychologically, the diaphragm area, at the base and center of the ribs, is the seat of the ego and houses our sense of outer-directed power. This area is symbolically related to external power, to how we present ourselves to the public, to our sense of self-confidence, and to our respect for ourselves as well as for others. Psychological associations are self-confidence, respect for self and others, and relationships to fear and external power. Since fear undermines self-confident presentation, a meditation on trust (see p. 77) focuses on calming anxieties and nurturing a sense of inner strength and confidence.

Third Chakra Meditation

Sit cross-legged or in a comfortable half-lotus position on a mat on the floor. Place a candle in front of you on a low table or chair so that the top of the candle is level with your eyes as you sit. Light the candle. Circle your thumbs to your forefingers and rest each hand, palm up, on your knees. Gaze steadily at the flame without blinking for about one minute. Then close your eyes, relax the muscles, and visualize an orange flame glowing between your eyebrows.

Alternate periods of flame-gazing with open eyes and flame-visualizing with closed eyes for periods of up to three minutes. Develop your gaze gradually. Do not strain your eyes. This sequence builds concentration and strengthens the nerve centers.

The positive always defeats the negative. Courage overcomes fear. Patience overcomes anger. Love overcomes hatred.

— Swami Sivananda Sarasvati

Each time you meditate, you may focus on one aspect of your emotional issues related to the powers of this body area, such as trust and self-confidence. Allow your thoughts to surface and then dissolve. Try to end your meditation with a feeling that encourages you to live more fully today. Visualize a warm orange-gold light inside your chest at the center base of your ribs. Allow the light to grow stronger.

Third Chakra Stretch Tips

- Breathe normally as you move. Do not hold your breath.

- Maintain a steady, controlled, slow pace during each exercise. Keeping control of the tempo helps build muscle, burn fat, and prevent injury.

- Always alternate a backward-motion exercise with a forward-motion one to balance muscle development and increase flexibility.

- Remember the Rush Reverse (see p. 36): reverse stretching can help you increase your flexibility and range of motion, and it can be applied to any movement, small and simple or long and complex.

Aromatherapy

Aromatherapy essential oils that help heal disorders of the third chakra area include cypress, vetiver, mimosa, damask rose, and jasmine. Italian cypress helps strengthen the functioning of the liver and the respiratory system, increases circulation, and calms nervous tension. Jasmine is soothing to the liver and the skin and is traditionally thought to promote feelings of optimism and confidence.

Third Chakra Stretches

⚷ COW-CAT

These exercises focus on your lower back muscles.

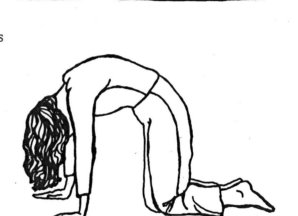

1. For the basic Cow-Cat, start on your hands and knees and then inhale as you look up at the ceiling, let your middle and lower back sink toward the floor, and arch your pelvis upward (the cow) — all at the same time.

2. As you exhale, curl your head and neck forward, tuck your pelvis under, and arch your middle back toward the ceiling in one fluid motion, like a stretching cat.

3. Alternate these positions as you inhale and exhale. Make the movements smooth and continuous.

This variation of the Cow-Cat incorporates balanced spinal movement.

1. Beginning on your hands and knees, inhale and extend your left leg behind you. You can stretch your right arm in front of you for extra balance practice, if comfortable.

2. Now exhale as you bend your left knee and bring the knee toward your chest, curling your neck forward and bringing your nose as far toward your knee as you can.

3. Next extend your left leg back, at the same time raising your right arm off the ground in front of you.

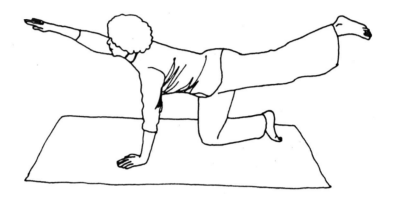

4. Then relax on your hands and knees.

5. Now try the same sequence with the other leg.

Another variation of the Cow-Cat helps ward off middle and lower back problems.

1. Kneel on your hands and knees with your head and neck relaxed forward and your pelvis tucked under.

2. Alternate moving your pelvis from side to side (left to right) with making full circles with your pelvis in both directions.

FISH

This exercise is a deeply relaxing stretch for the diaphragm, for the cervical and lumbar regions, and for the shoulders. The pose improves circulation to these areas and strengthens the thyroid and parathyroid. Breathe deeply through your nose. This can help relieve asthma or bronchial stress.

1. Either sit on the floor with your legs loosely crossed or kneel with your legs tucked under you, whichever is more comfortable. Different leg muscles will be toned. Lean back onto your forearms. Allow your weight to rest on your elbows as you arch your head and neck backward.

2. Slowly slide your elbows out from under you until the tip-top (not back) of your head is resting on the floor and your back is arched. Your arms are now free either to rest at your sides or to be raised over your head to stretch your legs and chest even more.

3. Inhale through your nose as you lift your arms above your head. Lie flat for a fuller stretch. Exhale as you bring your arms back to your sides. Alternate arm positions with your breathing. Unroll the pose slowly.

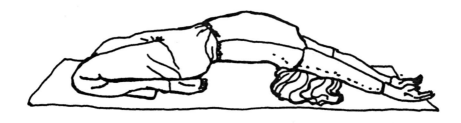

⚷ TRIANGLE TILT

This pose stretches your trunk muscles and spine. It improves flexibility of the hips, legs, and shoulders.

1. Stand straight, arms at your sides, palms on outer thighs, feet just more than shoulder width apart. A wider placement gives less stretch to your waist but may be more comfortable.

2. Inhale and raise one arm to the side, palm facing front.

3. Keeping your knees straight, exhale as you bend to the side over your lowered arm and stretch your upper arm to the side above your head, perpendicular to the floor. Your neck stays in a straight line with your spine, almost parallel to the floor. Turn your face up so that you can look at your raised hand.

4. Slide your lower hand toward your ankle. Be careful to bend sideways rather than forward. Hold this pose from a few seconds to a few minutes. Breathe through your nose.

5. Inhale as you straighten up slowly. Then try the pose to the opposite side.

✎ THE TWIST

This movement helps open up the muscles around the rib cage and the area around the diaphragm, which can be difficult to relax yet important because the diaphragm is the center of our breathing.

1. Place your feet farther apart than your shoulders, bend your knees, and squat slightly. Bend your arms at the elbows and rotate your hips in one direction as you move your shoulders in the other while facing forward. It's like dancing the twist.

2. Inhale as you twist to one side and exhale as you twist to the other. Do this movement a few times. When you're rocking on your feet, your knees will rotate from side to side, too.

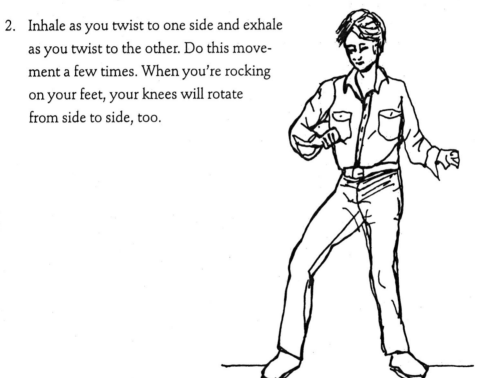

CROSS STRETCH

This movement stretches your groin muscles and tightens your waist.

1. Spread your feet wider apart than your shoulders, keeping your pelvis tucked under. Inhale. Spread both arms out to the side. Exhale as you lean to your left and touch near your left foot with the fingertips of your right hand.

2. Inhale as you stand up again.

3. Next exhale, lean over, and touch near your right foot with the fingertips of your left hand. While you're doing this exercise, make sure your head and neck are relaxed forward, so that you're not straining by holding up your head and looking up. You should be looking down at your toes and breathing as you move. If it's difficult for you to touch near your toes, help yourself by bending your knees more. Gradually the movement will become comfortable, and you will be able to do it with your knees just slightly bent.

FLOOR PATS

This stretches your back and waist.

1. Stand facing forward with your legs shoulder width apart. Look to your right as you turn your right foot outward and lean your torso to the right. Bend your right knee as deeply as is comfortable. Stretch your left leg out to the left and raise your left arm parallel to the floor.

2. Keep your head up as you bring your left palm down to touch the floor in front of your right foot.

3. Stand up and return to center. Reverse the position and repeat the movement on the other side.

Alternate right and left Floor Pats. Stand up in the center in between each. Try to make the movement smooth. If you do this exercise slowly, hold the stretch for a while. If you want to do it faster, just tap the floor and return to center. Inhale as you reach out and up. Exhale as you bend over and down.

CAMEL

This stretch opens your diaphragm.

1. Kneel and then sit back on your heels. Inhale as your raise your thighs and torso straight up over your knees. Allow your neck to arch back as you grasp your heels with your hands.

2. Exhale as you arch your back and neck more to increase the stretch. Hold this pose and breathe normally through your nose.

3. To unwind, exhale as you lower your chin toward your chest, straighten your back, and sit down on your shins.

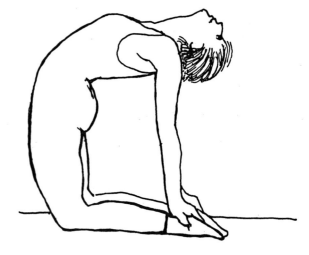

4. Now rest your back by leaning your torso forward onto your thighs and your forehead on the floor; relax your arms beside your legs.

COUNTING BREATHS

This simple meditation can be one of the most powerful.

1. Sit on the floor, spine erect, in a comfortable position. Close your eyes and place your hands, palms up, on your knees. Relax your breathing so you feel muscle movement low in your abdomen rather than high in your chest.

2. Begin counting your breaths. Count an inhalation plus an exhalation as one cycle; the next inhalation and exhalation is number two, and so on. Try to hold this focus without being sidetracked by other thoughts until you reach number ten.

3. If you got there without your mind wandering or losing count, you're probably an enlightened monk. At ten, start over with one and count ten breaths again. Continue this cycle for a minimum of ten minutes. Work up to longer sessions.

4. A significant weeding out of mental static is going on as you count and concentrate. It can be helpful to imagine the thoughts moving across a film screen, passing into and out of view. Try not to linger with the thoughts. Just notice them, let them pass, and return to counting breaths. Gradually, the thoughts will be spaced farther apart, and the periods of neutral focus will grow longer. Don't judge the content. We all have a thousand ways to distract ourselves from our deeper purpose.

5. After a while you may notice that when you're relaxed you pause at the end of your exhalation. Enjoy this and allow it to lengthen. Thoughts will become less frequent as you focus your attention on the slow exhalation and gentle pause.

SLOW ALTERNATE BREATH

1. Sit comfortably on the floor with the tip of your spine on a small pillow. Keep your legs crossed in front of you. Raise your right hand so the palm is toward your face. Specific fingers are used because of their differing magnetic charges. Fold down your index finger and the middle finger.

2. Press your thumb to close your right nostril and inhale with your left nostril to a count of four. Exhale to a count of eight. The exhalation should take twice as long as the inhalation.

3. Now release your thumb and press your left nostril closed with your ring and little fingers as you inhale through your right nostril to a count of four. Then exhale to a count of eight.

4. Continue this pattern of breathing for several cycles.

DOUBLE LOTUS

Sit back to back with your partner. Meditate together and notice how touching another person affects your awareness of your breathing. See if you can maintain your individual breath pattern even while sensing your partner's. Then match your breath rhythm to your partner's. Which way relaxes you more?

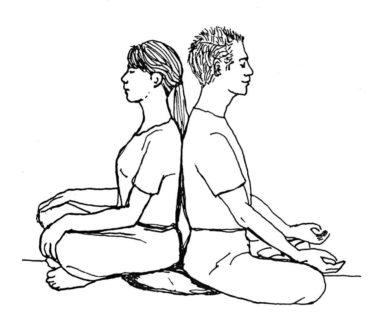

DOUBLED SIDE STRETCH

1. To give the muscles along your side great extension, sit on the floor with one leg bent and the foot tucked near the groin. The other leg is stretched out to your side. Your partner, sitting a leg's length to your side and facing the opposite way, does the same. The soles of your feet should meet. Inhale as you reach both arms over your head.

2. Then exhale as you tilt your torsos to the side toward each other and stretch over your extended legs. Clasp each other's extended hand. Allow your other arm to rest loosely on the floor in front of you. Stretch your side and tilt your head so that you are facing front but leaning to the side, not forward.

3. Breathe normally and relax in this position for a minute or two. Release slowly. Switch positions and repeat the posture in reverse to stretch your opposite legs and arms.

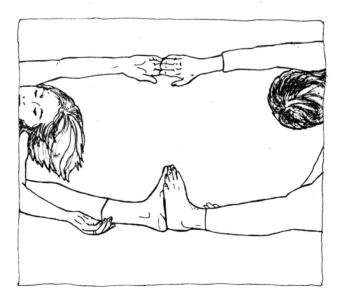

FOURTH CHAKRA STRETCH AREA
Chest, Mid-Back

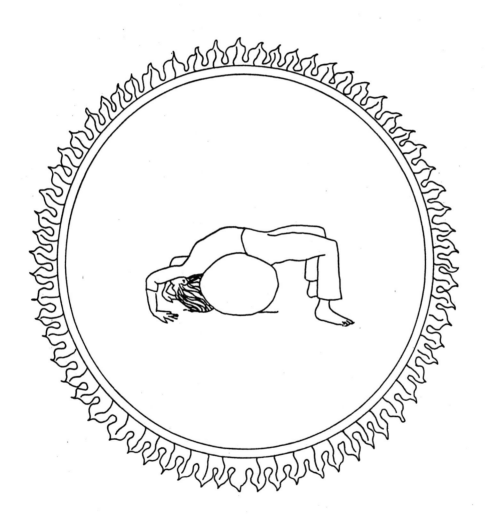

The cardiac nerve center of the fourth chakra area is centered in the chest and mid-back and includes the heart, the circulatory system, the thymus gland, and the thoracic vertebrae. A four-chambered heart is characteristic of all mammals. Every heartbeat sends out electrical impulses. A normal heartbeat lasts one second. The normal adult heart rate is between 60 and 80 beats per minute. A newborn's heart rate is about 150 beats per minute. Your circulatory system has two major jobs: transportation of materials and regulation of temperature.

Mind-Body Connection

If you understand the psychological connections of a body part, you can increase flexibility exercises for the area to relax emotional as well as physical tension. You can also explore these connections as you meditate.

The heart is the physical center of blood circulation for the body and is the psychological center of emotional attachment. The heart was the only organ not removed from a mummy by Egyptian embalmers because it was regarded as indispensable in the afterlife. Aristotle asserted that the heart, not the brain, was the seat of intelligence and sensation. A painting of a heart with flames symbolizes love as the center of spiritual illumination. Because blood represents life, spilled blood represents the sacrifice of life. The heart is the center of passion, which, when infused with enlightened understanding, becomes compassion, or love for others. Emotional associations are hope, forgiveness, hate, and love.

> *Someday, after we have mastered the winds, the waves, the tides, and gravity, we shall harness the engines of love. Then, for the second time in the history of the world, men will have discovered fire.*
>
> — Pierre Teilhard de Chardin

Fourth Chakra Meditation

You may light a candle or heat an essential oil incense with one of the healing scents for this chakra. Sit comfortably. Relax your breathing low in your abdomen. Silently ask how you can nourish your love and compassion.

Fourth Chakra Stretch Tips

- Breathe normally as you move. Do not hold your breath.

- It is important to lift your chest without straining your back and shoulders. Think of a rolltop desk and imagine you can roll your chest and upper back over your diaphragm as you slightly arch your lower back and inhale. Or try imagining that your head and neck are held upright by a string from above your head. This allows your chest and shoulders to relax downward.

- Remember the Rush Reverse (see p. 36): reverse stretching can help you increase your flexibility and range of motion, and it can be applied to any movement, small and simple or long and complex.

Aromatherapy

Aromatherapy essential oils that help heal disorders of the fourth chakra area include white birch, violet, damask rose, jasmine, longleaf pine, and lime. The scent of violets is traditionally believed to strengthen and comfort the heart. It relieves nervousness and insomnia and improves circulation. The oil has mild painkilling properties, which are attributed to the presence of salicylic acid, the active ingredient in aspirin. Damask rose improves circulation and relieves stress and is traditionally thought to be the scent of happiness.

Fourth Chakra Stretches

⚷ WING BACK STRETCH

This exercise helps open up your chest, helps relieve neck and upper-back tension, and makes your shoulder muscles more flexible.

1. Kneel on a mat with arms extended overhead and palms facing in toward each other. Tighten your stomach muscles by drawing your navel toward your spine as you exhale.

2. Releasing at your shoulder sockets, raise your arms higher as you inhale and lift your chest as you look up. Hold for two seconds; rest for five.

3. Repeat sequence.

4. Kneel and place a pillow about three feet in front of you. Clasp your arms behind you and rest them on your lower back.

5. As you exhale, gradually lean forward to touch your forehead to the pillow while you bring your clasped arms up behind you, pointing them toward the ceiling.

6. Reverse the motion and relax.

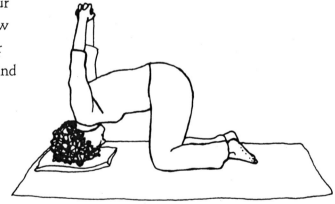

⚷ SPINAL TWIST

Any approximate position of this posture is good for the spine. You will gradually be able to twist all the way back.

1. Sit on the floor with your bent knees drawn up in front of your chest and your feet flat on the floor. Now allow your left knee to relax outward and draw the heel toward the crotch, allowing your knee to rest on the floor.

2. Cross your right foot over the left knee so it rests flat to the left side of the left knee. Slide your left foot to the outside of your right hip.

3. With the left hand, grasp the arch of the left foot. Do this by placing the arm on either the right or the left side of the right knee, whichever is comfortable.

4. Now look to your right and behind you as you wrap your right arm behind your back or rest it on the floor for support.

5. Continue to reach your right arm behind you, toward your right thigh or hip. Hold your chest erect. Use the leverage of the position to twist your spine backward.

6. Slowly unwind one limb at a time. Repeat this sequence with the reverse arm and leg.

⚷ TORSO HANG

Use this simple exercise to relax tight back muscles.

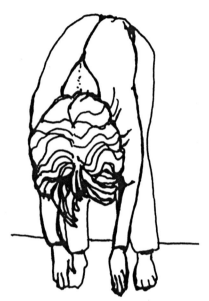

1. Standing, spread your feet about hip width apart. Relax your head and neck forward. Then slowly, vertebra by vertebra, curl your spine forward so that your arms are relaxed in front of you, reaching toward the floor.

2. Keep your knees slightly bent and try to touch the floor with your fingertips, but don't strain. Don't stretch, pull, or push your muscles. If you're not comfortable touching the floor, just approximate the position. You can allow your arms to swing gently while you hang to loosen your back as you breathe.

⚷ THE ARCH

This is one of my favorites, but if you've had any kind of back injury, you probably shouldn't attempt it. If you do have a healthy spine, doing this exercise is a good way to keep yourself limber and to balance out the more frequent forward movements that you make during the day.

1. Lie flat on your back. Bend your knees and draw your feet as close to your buttocks as possible. Then stretch your arms behind your head and place your palms on the floor with your elbows bent up toward the ceiling.

2. Pressing your feet down on the floor, inhale and raise your pelvis off the floor.

3. Gradually arch your whole back, pushing up with your hands and feet. Breathe in this position a few seconds.

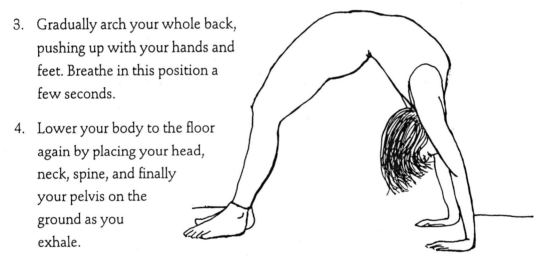

4. Lower your body to the floor again by placing your head, neck, spine, and finally your pelvis on the ground as you exhale.

5. Bring your bent knees up over your chest and rest a few moments on your back in this position.

THE ARCH VARIATION

Before you have built enough muscle strength to do the Arch, you can lie backward over a large exercise ball to release tension in the chest and upper back.

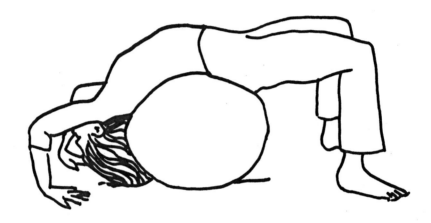

CRACKING YOUR BACK

You might want to try "cracking" your spine to release tension in your back muscles. One easy way to do that is to incorporate it into an exercise called the Hip Fold. While lying down, move your knees together from side to side on the floor. Twist your spine more and try to use the weight of your legs to "crack" your spine as you roll your hips.

You can also try cracking your back from a standing squat. It took me several weeks of doing this motion gently once or twice every day before my spine finally "cracked." Once it did, I had the feel for it; now I can do it easily at any time. Persist!

1. Spread your legs wide apart, bend your knees, and hunch over with your palms on your knees so that your shoulders are up toward your ears and your body weight rests on your hands and arms.

2. Keep your spine and torso facing forward, but as you exhale, twist your right shoulder toward your left side so that you can feel a slight pull in your lower spine.

3. Try the same motion with your left shoulder, moving it toward your right side, feeling your vertebrae curl.

BOW

1. To open your chest and mid-back areas, lie flat with your forehead on the floor. Bend your knees and reach behind you to grasp both ankles.

2. With arms straight, inhale and raise your head, chest, and legs to form a backward arch with your whole body. The stretch comes from trying to straighten your legs and torso while still clasping your ankles.

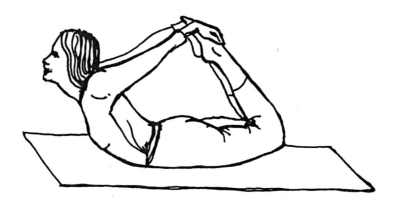

3. Breathe normally and hold the pose for up to thirty seconds. Exhale as you slowly release the pose and lie down.

A variation for more stretch is to inhale and rock back, then exhale and rock forward as you hold your ankles.

LYING ARM STRETCH

This exercise improves the range of motion in your shoulders.

1. Lie on the floor on your back. Bend your knees, keeping your feet flat on the floor. Raise your right hand over your head and place your palm on the floor behind you. Stretch your extended arm behind your head as far as you can, inhaling as you do so.

2. Stretch the arm resting at your side toward your feet, so that your arms are stretching in opposite directions. Notice how this opens up muscles in your back that you don't often release. Hold that position for several seconds and then relax.

3. Reverse the position and repeat the movement.

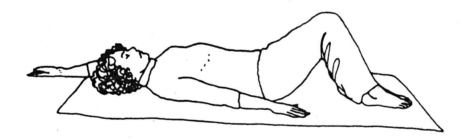

Rests

When you feel that your back is strained, even slightly, or that you need to rest for a little while to regain some energy, there are several restorative positions you can use.

One is to lie on your side and draw your knees toward your chest, keeping your head and your spine in a straight line and folding your arms across your chest.

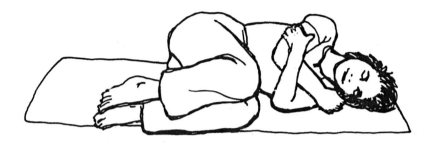

This next position for resting the spine is more comfortable for some people than for others. Kneel, sitting on your heels, and arch your back slightly. Lower the front of your head to the floor. Let both arms hang loosely at your sides, palms up, and see if you can really release your shoulders, so that they're hanging toward the floor. Take several deep breaths, so that your whole spine and back open up as you sit in this position.

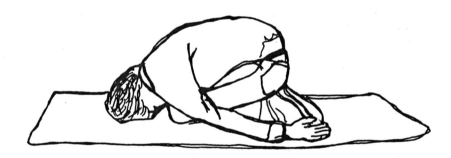

You can use these rest positions in between exercises, to break from any strenuous activity, or at any moment when you feel the need to relax. It's an important part of preventive exercise to assume these relaxing positions from time to time and to treat yourself kindly so that you never overstress.

TWO CIRCLING

This exercise stretches the muscles of your back.

1. Sit on the floor facing your partner. Spread your legs comfortably. Hold hands with your partner and keep the soles of your feet together.

2. Begin with one person leaning forward while the other leans back, supporting each other with your hands and feet.

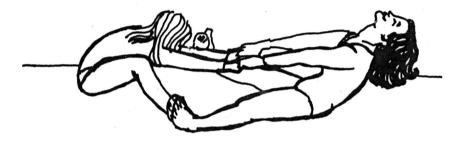

3. Gradually change your forward motion to a sideways motion so that you both begin to draw large circles on the floor with the movement of your torsos.

4. Inhale and lean back and to the right.

5. Lean your torso farther to the right as you lean forward; then come to the center.

6. Now make a larger circle, moving your head and torso to the left.

Increase the speed of your circling as much as is comfortable. Keep your breathing synchronized so that you inhale as you arch backward and exhale as you drop forward. Going faster and faster can be fun if the position is physically comfortable.

BACK BREATHING FOR TWO

This exercise enables two people to tune in to their own backs and their partner's as well.

1. Sit back to back on the floor with your legs crossed. Relax your hands in your lap and close your eyes. Without talking, try to arrange your body positions so you can comfortably lean on each other with mutual support and no strain.

2. Once you've found this position together, tune in to your own breathing and try to relax the rest of your body so that the breath moves deep in your belly. Note the muscles of your back that move in response to your breathing. Notice your partner's back and how it feels leaning against you. See if you can feel the movement of your partner's muscles in his/her back as a result of breathing.

3. Once you have tuned in to your partner's breathing, notice whether you change your own breathing while searching for your partner's. Did you change your breath pattern to match your partner's without thinking? If such changes happen, see whether you can let your breath relax in your belly again and maintain your own rhythm while being aware of your partner's. The ability to do this is often related to your patterns in daily relationships and the capability of being sensitive to another person's habits while maintaining your own.

4. A good way to end this exercise is to imagine that you are each exhaling through your lower back, as though you could breathe into each other's backs. Let yourself do this awhile and see what sensations arise. Now lock arms at the elbows. Place your feet flat on the floor with your knees bent. See if you can help each other stand up back to back!

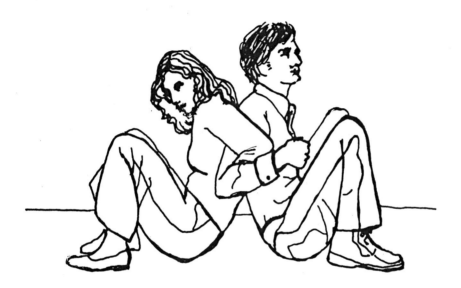

FIFTH CHAKRA STRETCH AREA
Shoulders, Upper Back,
Base of Neck, Arms, Hands

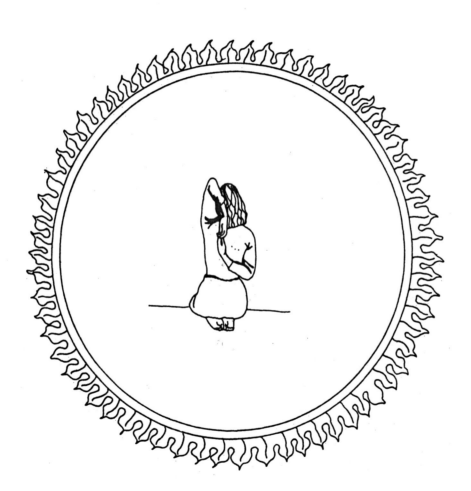

The nerve center of the fifth chakra is focused in the throat area and includes the base of the neck, the upper shoulders, the arms and hands, and the nerves and body chemicals that guide impulses through this area. Eight pairs of cervical nerves control your neck and arms. One fingertip contains three thousand touch receptors. Touch stimulates the brain's production of natural pain suppressors.

Mind-Body Connection

If you understand the psychological connections of a body part, you can increase flexibility exercises for the area to relax emotional as well as physical tension. You can also explore these connections as you meditate.

Psychologically, the throat is the center of communication. The mouth is viewed as a kind of doorway through which our inner thoughts can cross to the outside world. Because speech is produced from air coming out of our mouths, the mouth is symbolic of creating something from nothing. In many spiritual traditions, a word is thought to have been the first creation of God and, therefore, is symbolic of original divine creation. Thus, singing is considered a holy part of religious ritual.

Arms and hands can make things, build things, harm or shield things. They are symbolically linked to the throat by their function for external creation. Because of the hands' role in work, they are a symbol of action in the exterior world. A closed fist symbolizes defense or attacks. An open hand symbolizes creation, receptivity, and healing. Psychological associations are the ability to make decisions, to be aggressive, and to create.

> *May I help all beings.*
>
> — Avalokiteshvara,
> Buddha of Compassion

Fifth Chakra Meditation

Sit on a mat on the floor with a small pillow under your tailbone for support. Relax your hands, palms up, on your knees. Circle each thumb to its forefinger. Repeat the following breathing sequence ten times to relax the throat area, and clear the lungs by lengthening the exhalation.

With your mouth closed, slightly tighten and close the back of your throat as you inhale through your nose, so that you produce a light snoring sound.

With your mouth still closed, exhale slowly through your nose as you produce a low humming sound in your throat. You may imagine that your throat is bathed in a pale blue light.

As you meditate, you may focus on aspects of your emotional issues related to the powers of this body area, such as communication and creative work. Allow thoughts to surface, be noted, and dissolve with your exhalations.

Fifth Chakra Stretch Tips

- Breathe normally as you move. Do not hold your breath.

- Keep your jaw relaxed while you exercise. Jaw clenching can cause headaches and shoulder aches.

- When bending forward, do not drop your shoulders first; this hurts your back. Bend fully forward from your hip joints. Keep chin tucked under.

- If your jaw makes a clicking sound as you move it, see your dentist to check whether you have TMJ problems.

- Remember the Rush Reverse (see p. 36): reverse stretching can help you increase your flexibility and range of motion, and it can be applied to any movement, small and simple or long and complex.

Aromatherapy

Essential oils that especially nurture the fifth chakra system include East Indian sandalwood, spearmint, Canadian balsam, sweet orange, frankincense, and Roman chamomile. Breathing the scents of sandalwood and Canadian balsam helps clear the sinuses and throat. White birch has a bracing scent that encourages calm confidence. Sweet orange blossom scent encourages emotional balance.

Fifth Chakra Stretches

FAN CIRCLES

Relaxing your hands will release nervous tension in your body and maintain good circulation in your wrists and fingers. In yoga, each posture is designed to focus electromagnetic and nerve currents in different parts of the body. The hands and feet are directional pointers, or turn signals, in the body's circuitry. Experiment with making free-form movements and circles in as many ways and directions as you can with your hands and wrists, spreading, opening, and closing your fingers like a fan as you do.

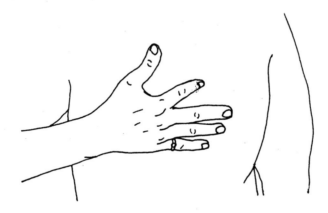

UPPER-BACK WING FOLDS

This motion helps relax neck and shoulder tension, especially between your shoulder blades.

1. Lie on your back on a firm bed or a mat on the floor. Rest your arms just below shoulder height at your sides. Bend your knees. Position your head, spine, and hips in a straight line. Notice where you feel your spine touching the ground or bed and where you feel it held away. Feel the weight of your head on the floor or bed.

2. As you inhale, gently roll your head to the right side as far as you can without any muscle resistance in your neck or shoulders. This may be only a few inches. Exhale as you roll your head back to center.

3. Rest a breath in the center without moving.

4. Then roll your head to the left as you inhale, only as far as is easy with no resistance. Exhale as you roll your head back to center. Rest a breath in the center without moving.

5. Now include your arms in the movement. Stretch your right arm out to the right. Inhale as you roll your head to the right and also fold your left arm over your chest. Lift the left arm at the shoulder joint. Your left hand will lightly touch your right arm as you fold. Try to keep the hands just below shoulder height to avoid back tension.

6. As you move your arms, notice where the movement begins: in the muscles on either side of the spine between the shoulder blades.

7. Roll your left arm and your head back to center. Rest a breath here.

8. Stretch your left arm out to the left as you inhale and fold your right arm over your chest.

9. Exhale as you roll both back to center.

10. Continue this side-to-side motion gently, slowly, and smoothly.

11. Rest in the center without moving. Notice how your spine is lying on the ground or bed. Is any more of your spine or neck touching than when you began? If so, this means that your motion has relaxed the muscles' cramping, and they have lengthened. Try the head roll by itself. Can you move farther to each side without strain than when you began?

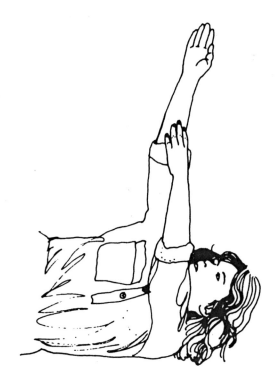

LYING UPPER-BACK RELEASE

This exercise reaches the upper back and neck, which are difficult to exercise and are usually quite tense. The hip joints, parts of the buttocks, and the lower back also benefit from these movements.

1. Lie on your back; bend your knees and draw both legs up to your chest. Prop yourself on your elbows so that your knees come toward your forehead. Don't strain; just relax in this position.

2. Now let your head and neck relax backward gradually and sink between your shoulders so that your shoulders are hunched up. Allow gravity to pull your head backward.

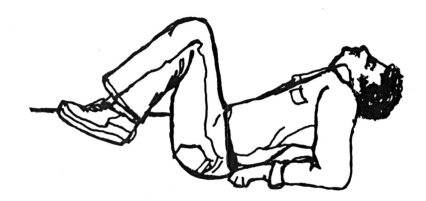

3. Next let both knees roll sideways. Rotate both legs from side to side, moving your knees toward the floor and rolling your hips on the floor. Inhale as you bring your knees toward the center; exhale as you move your knees to one side.

4. Next add a rotation of your head from side to side. Try moving your head in the same direction that you're rotating your knees and sometimes in the opposite direction.

5. Also try moving your shoulders around while your head is resting backward. In this way you can massage the trapezius and upper back muscles that are often difficult to reach. Do these rotations very slowly, but be sure to let the weight of your legs carry your knees all the way to the floor and give your spine a good, slow, rolling stretch from both ends.

6. End by bringing your knees back to center, keeping your back relaxed and your head sunk between your shoulders.

7. Exhale as you raise your neck and bring your forehead toward your knees.

8. Inhale as you relax your whole torso and lower your legs onto the floor.

9. Lie flat and rest.

⚷ HOLDING HANDS

This exercise opens up the chest and helps release the upper-back and shoulder tension that many of us have. It may be done while standing, sitting, or kneeling.

1. Inhaling, raise your left arm. Then place your left palm behind your upper back as you point your left elbow toward the ceiling. Position your palm over your spine between the shoulder blades.

2. Bend your right arm at the elbow, tucking your hand under you, and bring your right arm up behind you, sliding the back of your right hand up your spine to meet your left palm.

3. Hold hands with yourself behind your back. (If you can't touch or hold your hands, don't worry: it will come with practice. Just hold the position as close as you can.) Breathe and relax in this position for a few seconds.

4. Release the position slowly.

5. Now reverse the position of your arms to repeat the same motion on the other side.

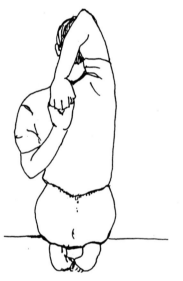

NECK ROLLS

These moves relax the muscles of the neck, shoulders, and upper chest.

Sitting

Sit comfortably and relax your head forward. Then make slow circles with your head from right to left. Next circle left to right. Be careful not to tilt the head too far backward as this can pinch a nerve in your neck.

Left

1. Stand with your feet about shoulder width apart. Look forward. Inhale as you raise both arms, palms up, from your sides. Straighten your spine, keeping your chest high and your lower back relaxed. Bring your palms together centered over your head.

2. Exhale as you turn your head left toward your left shoulder. Keep your elbows pressed back, in line with your shoulders.

3. Inhale as you roll your head back and allow your neck to relax so your head falls as far back onto your upper back as is comfortable. Exhale as you roll your head and neck toward the right shoulder.

Right

4. Inhale as you raise your head up so that you are looking toward your right shoulder.

5. Exhale and bring your head facing forward. Try to keep your shoulders pressed back and your body relaxed while you perform the head rolls.

6. To start another rotation, allow your head and neck to relax forward so you stretch the back of your neck in a new direction. Then roll your head to the left again. Perform three or four left head rolls.

7. Repeat this whole sequence moving your head in the opposite direction; circle right to left several times.

8. Roll very slowly to begin. Gradually speed up the pace only if you can comfortably maintain very smooth movement in your neck.

SHOULDER SNAKES

This motion relaxes tight trapezius muscles in the shoulders and can be done while sitting or standing.

1. Bend your elbows close to your sides with wrists raised to a height just below your shoulders. Press both shoulders down slightly.

2. Keeping your head and neck upright, draw both shoulders backward.

3. Now raise both shoulders up toward your ears.

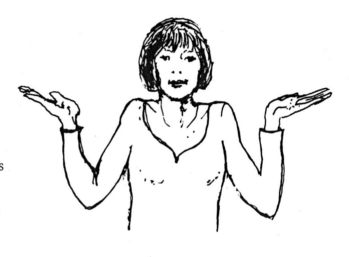

4. Allow your shoulders to relax forward and down. Repeat this cycle three or four times. Try to allow your movement to be smooth and continuous rather than jerky.

5. Do this movement in the opposite direction so that your shoulders roll first up and back, then down and forward.

For more precise flexibility, you can snake each shoulder separately.

SHOULDER JOGS

You can feel that this motion limbers the muscles around your shoulder blades.

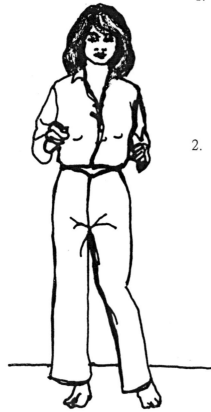

1. Standing, bend your arms at the elbows and bring one arm forward while the other goes back. Move at the shoulder as though you were jogging, but move only your arms. Move with your breathing so that you inhale as one arm goes back and exhale as it comes forward.

2. Next, while bending your arms at the elbows stand in a comfortable position. Bring your elbows out to the side, up toward the ceiling. Now raise one elbow higher as you lower the other. Check your knees to be sure that they are gently bent and that your legs are comfortable.

STANDING UPPER-BACK OPENER

1. Stand with one foot about twelve inches in front of you, your hands clasped behind you. Keep your rear leg straight.

2. Inhale as you lean your head and torso over your knee and bend the forward leg. As you lean forward, raise your clasped arms behind you.

3. Stretch your arms upward so you can feel your shoulder pockets opening and your shoulder blades moving toward each other.

4. Exhale as you lower your arms and stand up straight again.

5. Now bring the back leg forward and repeat this motion bending your other leg.

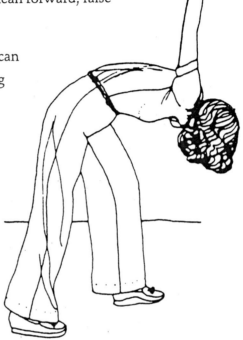

STANDING SQUAT

Squatting keeps your knees, thighs, and other leg muscles strong and keeps all the joints in your legs and hips limber, so that you can stand and lift using your leg muscles rather than your back muscles. A variation of the floor squat is the Standing Squat.

1. Hold on to the edge of a counter, strong chair, or table that's waist height. Begin a movement cycle so that you inhale as you stand up and exhale as you squat. Keep your back straight and your pelvis tucked under. Be sure not to arch your back. Keep your heels flat on the floor for as long as possible while you're squatting, raising them only when your hips get close to the floor.

2. Sit on your heels and rest in that position for a few seconds.

3. Now inhale and stand up. This is also a good shoulder and upper-back release.

THE PIANO

The best limbering you could give your hands is to learn to play the harp or piano. Short of that, try this exercise that you can do anywhere.

1. Rest your palms on your lap or a table. One by one, raise and then press down with each finger of the left hand in sequence.

2. Repeat with the fingers of the right hand.

3. Now, slowly enough so that you do not skip any fingers touching down, do the exercise with both hands at once.

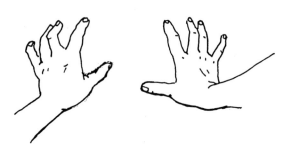

MOON RISE

This movement sequence stretches almost all your muscles in almost every direction as you and your partner move. The steps are described separately but should be performed simultaneously so they form a complete sweeping and turning motion.

Beginning

1. Stand facing each other, arm's length apart, and clasp hands between you. Tilt your pelvis forward and relax your chest.

2. Shift your weight so you are standing on your outside leg (the man's right, the woman's left in this illustration).

Moon Rise

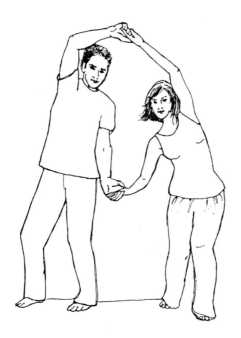

3. Raise your outside arm (the man's right, the woman's left) high over your head as you lower your inside arm.

4. At the same time, turn your torso and head forward. The man turns to his right, the woman to her left. Also swing your inside leg forward between the two of you so you are both standing facing outward now.

Full Moon

5. Continue to turn in the same outward direction while keeping your hands clasped together.

6. End up back to back, arching backward and keeping your hands clasped. The palms are now facing up.

7. Raise your arms as high as is comfortable as you tilt your pelvis forward to accentuate the arch.

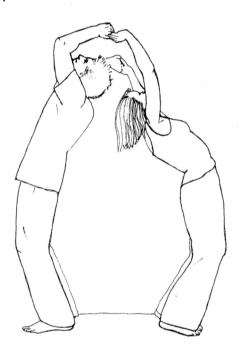

Moon Set

8. Continue to step and turn in the same direction while maintaining clasped hands.

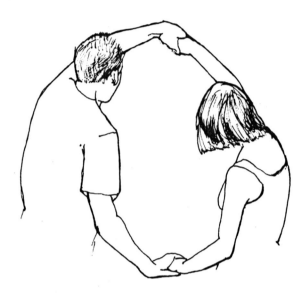

9. Roll down out of the arch by stepping to the opposite side (man to his right, woman to her left) until you have your outside arms (man's left, woman's right) overhead and your inside arms down at your sides between you.

10. Gradually complete the turn so that you come full circle back to your starting position, facing each other.

You can rest in the center a moment or you can keep moving so that you begin the Moon Rise all over again without pausing. Practice this slowly. Speed up the pace so that you can perform four full Moon Rises in a row.

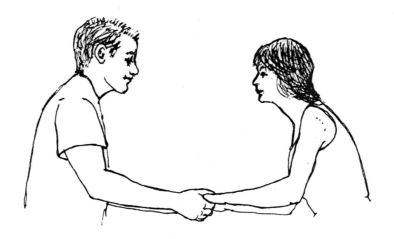

SIXTH CHAKRA STRETCH AREA
Face, Neck

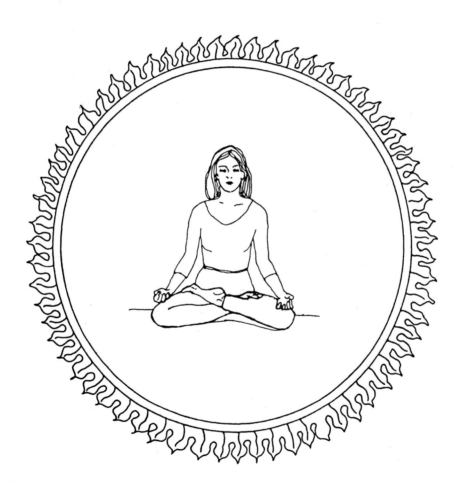

The forehead plexus, or the sixth chakra, encompasses the face, ears, and base of the skull, including the pineal gland, the nervous system, and the medulla of the brain. The necks of all mammals, no matter what size, are composed of seven vertebrae.

Mind-Body Connection

If you understand the psychological connections of a body part, you can increase flexibility exercises for the area to relax emotional as well as physical tension. You can also explore these connections as you meditate.

The eyes are associated with clarity of perception, of others as well as of oneself. They are connected with light and, thus, are a symbol of receiving and sending out light and can also signify intelligence and understanding. Since having two eyes is the human norm, many religious paintings show an extra eye in the center of the forehead to represent divine understanding. Eyes painted on other body parts depict the use of that part for high spiritual purposes. The face is the symbol of how we show ourselves to the world and of our ability to look at challenges with courage and honesty. Being "two-faced" means being dishonest. Emotional associations are courage, intelligence, and the ability to evaluate oneself and others.

Knowledge is the true organ of sight, not the eyes.

— Panchatantra, fifth-century Buddhist morality tales

Sixth Chakra Meditation

Sit in a comfortable lotus position on a mat on the floor. Place a small pillow under your tailbone. Relax your hands, palms up, on your knees. Circle each thumb to its forefinger.

Close your eyes. Turn your eyes up and focus them toward the space between the eyebrows. This is the location of the pituitary gland, or "third eye," which when stimulated increases intuition and clarity of thought. Directing your eye gaze at this point stimulates the olfactory nerves, optic nerves, and central nervous system. Start by holding this gaze for one to two minutes. Gradually increase to ten minutes, but no longer. Holding too long strains the eyes and nerves. However long you hold the gaze, spend the same amount of time afterward relaxing the eyes in a level position.

> *Who sees the divine amid the mortal,*
> *that man sees truly.*
> — Bhagavad Gita

Each time you meditate, you may focus on one aspect of your emotional issues related to the powers of this body area, such as honesty. Allow thoughts to surface and then dissolve.

As you meditate, imagine that a warm, golden light is glowing at the spot in the center of your forehead between your eyes.

Sixth Chakra Stretch Tips

- Breathe normally as you move. Do not hold your breath.

- Pushing a stretch too far (beyond your comfort level) leads to formation of scar tissue in the muscle and loss of elasticity.

- Closing your eyes while resting or stretching deepens the relaxation by encouraging alpha brain-wave states.

- Remember the Rush Reverse (see p. 36): reverse stretching can help you increase your flexibility and range of motion, and it can be applied to any movement, small and simple or long and complex.

Aromatherapy

Essential oils that help heal disorders of the sixth chakra area include cardamom, vetiver, coriander, spearmint, lavender vera, and damask rose. Add a few drops of cardamom oil to East Indian sandalwood oil for a heady meditation incense. Cardamom relieves nervous strain and mental fatigue. Indian sandalwood lifts depression and relieves insomnia and stress reactions. In Asia, sandalwood is a favorite building material for temples. Spearmint helps relieve sinusitis, headache, fatigue, and nervous strain. The oil is beneficial to the skin. The scent targets the head and sinus area.

Sixth Chakra Stretches

🔑 NECK AND TORSO RELEASE

This exercise — developed by Moshe Feldenkrais, a movement expert — improves flexibility in your neck, chest, and spine.

1. Sit on the front of a chair or stool, palms resting on thighs, feet flat on the floor and shoulder width apart. Making small, gentle movements, look to the right and turn your torso that way. Then slowly return to face forward. Notice how far you can turn without tension. Pause.

2. Next focus your eyes on a spot straight ahead and keep looking at this spot throughout this exercise. Exhale as you turn your head and torso to the right. Notice that you don't turn as far when you keep your gaze fixed straight ahead. Pause a moment.

3. Now repeat this turn to the right but turn your eye focus to the right also. You probably can turn farther this time. Return to center position. Then turn only your shoulders and chest to the right as your head and gaze remain forward. Notice that your left shoulder moves forward as your right moves back. Return to center. Pause.

4. Gently turn your eyes, head, and torso to the right. Return to center. Is turning becoming easier? Do you feel different on your right and left sides?

5. Keep your feet flat on the floor as you move your left knee forward. Your lower back, shoulders, and head will turn to the right a bit. Return to center. Move your left knee forward while turning your torso and head to the right. Do you feel that moving your knee helps you turn? Do you feel a little taller? Pause to rest.

6. Next, repeat the entire sequence of movements to the left.

7. Now alternate turning right and left a few times. Move slowly and smoothly. Notice if you feel more flexible.

8. Alternate turning your hips and torso to the right and left as your eyes and head are turning in the opposite direction. Pause.

9. Now move your left knee forward as you turn right. Then do the same to the left. Notice if your flexibility and range have increased without strain or stretch. How do you feel when you stand?

⚷ HEAD CRADLES

Center

This exercise helps release neck and upper-back tension. If done gently, it strengthens the muscles in the front and on the sides of your neck.

1. Lie on your back. Bend your knees. Bring your feet close to your buttocks. Relax your lower back flat on the floor. Extend your arms sideways on the floor, palms up. Relax your jaw and shoulders. Press your shoulder blades down. Lift your head about two inches and gently extend your neck longer. Lower your head to the floor.

2. Now slowly lift your head. Tuck in your chin, looking at the floor between your feet.

3. Reverse this motion slowly, allowing each neck vertebra to release down toward the floor separately. Allow your shoulders and arms to stay relaxed as you move your head. Rest your head, chin tucked in, down on the floor last.

Diagonal

1. In the same starting position as for the center Head Cradle, place both hands behind your head. Bend your elbows and point them toward the ceiling. Use your hands and arms (not your neck) to lift your head off the floor. Curl your neck and head forward so that your chin is angled toward your chest.

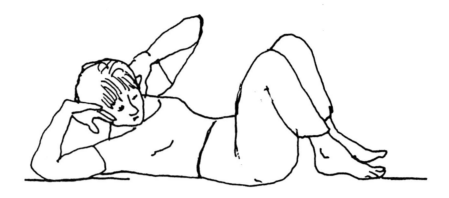

2. Now open your arms and place your hands beside your ears as you roll your head to each side several times. Try to touch each shoulder with your chin.

Stretching your neck and upper back this way will release deep neck tension if you do the exercise regularly and extremely gently.

🔑 HEAD ROLLS

This movement tones neck muscles and frees neck motion.

1. Sit with your spine erect, shoulders relaxed, and arms resting in your lap.

2. Slowly roll your head to one side, then down to the front, then to the other side, then backward. Allow the roll to be smooth and continuous.

3. Repeat the sequence several times. Notice where your motion catches.

4. Reverse the direction and roll your head to the other side.

CLOCK FACE

This exercise strengthens the eye muscles and improves the eyesight. Start with brief sessions and gradually increase the length.

1. Sit in a comfortable meditation pose with spine erect. Close your eyes.

2. Imagine your face has a clock painted on it. Keeping your eyelids closed, look up as far as you can at a spot in the center of your forehead where the number 12 would be on the clock. Hold this gaze for a count of five.

3. Shift your gaze a bit to the right as though you were looking at the number 1 on the clock, about the middle of your right eyebrow. Hold this gaze for five seconds.

4. Shift your gaze to the far corner of your right eye, where the number 2 would be. Hold the gaze for about five seconds.

5. Continue around your face in a clockwise direction, stopping at each imaginary number until you reach 12 again.

6. Then reverse the process and gaze at each number in a counterclockwise sequence. Rest a moment with closed eyes; then open them slowly.

NECK FLEXES

This helps correct a common tendency to carry the head forward and down so that the seven cervical (neck) vertebrae are out of line and the normal curve of the neck is exaggerated.

Center

1. Sit comfortably. Relax your facial muscles. Open your mouth slightly so that you won't clench your jaw. Now draw your chin in toward your neck as you extend your neck up as much as possible. Keeping the chin in allows you to use the inner neck muscles to balance your skull on top of the neck bones and to release tension in the base of the neck.

2. Curl your head down toward your chest and look toward your chin. Place one hand on the back top of your head and gently angle your head down, lengthening the muscles of the back of your neck and into the base of your skull. If you feel the stretch below your neck but not up into your head, your neck is too far forward.

3. Now turn your head a little to the right and hold this position for two seconds. Next, turn your head a little to your left and hold two seconds.

Side

1. Align your head vertically, as you did for the center Neck Flex.

2. Turn your head sideways to your right. Your ear is over your shoulder and your face looks forward, not down or up. Place your right hand on the left top side of your head. Gently angle your head toward your right shoulder. Hold this position for two seconds.

3. Relax your shoulders. Hold them down for two seconds.

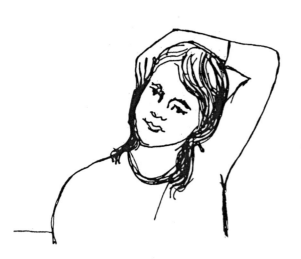

4. Reach toward the floor with your left arm to help you lengthen more in the neck muscles on your left side. Slowly reach a bit forward with your left arm. Then reach backward while still angling your arm down.

5. Using your left hand to lean your head to the left side, repeat this stretch to the left.

Diagonal

You will feel this stretch in your neck where the back and side meet.

1. Align your head vertically. Place your right hand on the back of the top of your head. Curve your head forward. Now move your head and neck on a diagonal toward your right knee. Next, turn your head to the left.

2. With your right hand on the left back of your head, gently angle your head downward. Hold this stretch for two seconds.

3. Reach your left arm behind you and pull it down toward the floor in a back diagonal and hold this position for two more seconds. Repeat the diagonal Neck Flex on your left side.

SIDE SHOULDER STRETCH

These shoulder muscle stretches are helpful to do before lifting weights or playing any sport. Anyone who uses his/her arms in a forward position at work can maintain flexibility and prevent stiffness and injury by using these stretches before and after work.

1. A seated position helps protect your lower back. You can sit on the floor, a chair, or a stool. Hold a towel in both hands, with your hands two to three feet apart. Raise your arms out in front of you, elbows relaxed.

2. Raise your arms over your head, back to the place just before where you feel tightness in the top front of your shoulder joint. Stop moving there.

3. Now move both arms and the towel to the right. Don't tilt your body. Moving the triangle of your arms and the towel sideways about six inches will stretch each shoulder.

4. Bend your right elbow and use your right hand to pull the left extended arm back below and behind its tight place. This gentle pull will stretch

the front top of your right shoulder muscles and the muscles between the shoulder blades. Hold the arm stretch for two seconds at a time.

5. Reverse this position by moving the arm triangle to your left and bending your left elbow. Use your left arm to pull your right extended arm back. You should feel this stretch in the front of your right shoulder muscles and between your shoulder blades. Hold this stretch for two seconds at a time.

6. Straighten your left arm. Return your arms above your head and then angle them completely back so that the towel is now behind your head. Move your arms slowly backward and down so that their final position is down at your sides, with the towel behind you. Release pose.

7. Now lie on your back on a bed, with your head at a corner of the foot of the bed. Hold the towel in front of you and raise your arms over your head. Gravity will pull the weight of your arms and help stretch your muscles enough for them to yield and move through their full range of motion. Try the side shoulder stretches in this position.

HANG LOOSE

This stretch helps loosen your neck and shoulders.

1. Sit on a chair and lean forward with your knees bent. Relax
    your spine and neck and let your arms hang toward the
    floor. It's important to keep your knees
    bent so that you don't strain your
    back. Be sure to let your neck
    fully relax. You can shake your
    head a few times. Let your
    arms hang. This position
    could be a warm-up for any
    exercise requiring touching
    your toes, but now you're
    simply relaxing.

2. Let your arms swing and rotate
    and feel how this gently opens your
    upper back around your shoulder blades.

Sitting from Reclining

This sequence helps prevent neck and upper-back strain. When lying on
your back, move to a sitting position by rolling onto your side, bending your
knees slightly while bringing them up toward your chest. Roll your weight
forward onto your arms and hands and push yourself up from your side to a
sitting position.

NECK HELP FOR TWO

1. In this exercise for double neck relaxation, one person stands while the other sits down, legs straight out, with his/her back to the partner's feet. The sitting person leans back against the legs of the stander.

2. If you are standing, bend your knees slightly; let your head relax forward; place your palms on either side of your friend's head. Gently move your friend's head from left to right. Ideally, the person sitting on the floor will relax enough so that when you are moving his/her head, he/she won't tense against the side-to-side movement.

3. Then help your partner relax her head forward.

4. If you are standing, next place one palm on your partner's head. If you are sitting on the floor, let your back relax and let your neck and head fall forward. Let your whole torso lean toward your legs as you exhale.

5. If you are standing, flex your knees gently to rock the person sitting in front of you. Don't push your friend any farther forward than is comfortable.

6. After a few minutes of rocking, slowly straighten your knees and let your friend sit up.

7. Place your palms around the back of the skull and let your fingers curl around either side of the jaw. Try raising your friend's head slightly so that you stretch the neck. If you are sitting down, relax and allow your head to be lifted. The stretching movement should be smooth and slight so that you do not strain the person's neck.

8. If you are standing, place your palms behind your friend's head and let him/her lean back to rest the whole head in your hands.

9. Now, holding your friend's head in your hands, walk backward and ease him/her down so that your friend can eventually come to a flat, resting position on the floor.

If you are lying down, relax for a while, noting the way your body feels from the exercise. Then trade places with your partner and repeat the exercise.

SEVENTH CHAKRA STRETCH AREA
Head, Mind

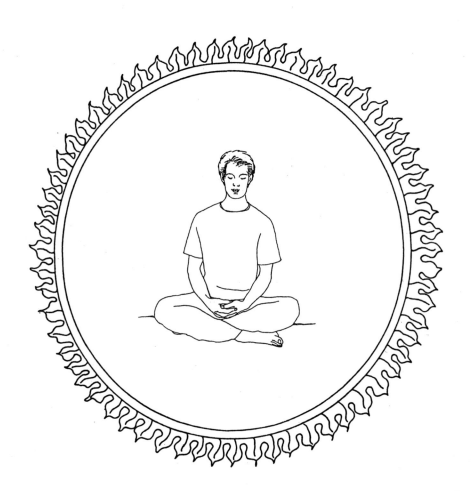

The cranial plexus of the seventh chakra is centered in the scalp and skull, including the pituitary gland and the cerebral cortex. The human head weighs between twelve and eighteen pounds, giving your neck quite a job to hold it up all day. Twelve pairs of cranial nerves control your head and its sense organs, as well as some autonomic reactions. The skull consists of eight bones joined together at the skull's immovable joints, or suture lines.

The brain needs twenty-five times as much oxygen as muscles do. Exercises can strengthen the neck muscles and improve the blood flow to your brain. Good circulation to your head not only stimulates your gray matter; it also improves the functioning of your whole body because the brain controls and orders your muscle activity. The brain is the boss.

Mind-Body Connection

If you understand the psychological connections of a body part, you can increase flexibility in the area by relaxing emotional as well as physical tension. Meditation helps you explore these connections.

The skull is the symbolic crown of the body, representing higher powers directed upward. Since the head is a sphere, it is a symbol of oneness and centeredness. The skull inside the head is symbolic of the inseparable cycle of death and life. Hair generally symbolizes energy; thus, cutting it represents losing vitality. Spiritually, cutting your own hair symbolizes intentionally giving up physical power for spiritual insight. This is the meaning of the practice of monks shaving their heads. The top of the head is symbolic of a person's connection to higher spiritual powers. Psychological associations include values, courage, and a sense of spiritual responsibility to others.

Seventh Chakra Meditation

Sit in a comfortable lotus position on a mat on the floor. Place a small pillow under your tailbone. Relax your hands, palms up, on your knees. Touch the thumb of each hand to the forefinger.

Our experience necessarily begins with direct reflection on . . . the many facets of impermanence.

— Sogyal Rinpoche

Close your eyes. Focus your attention on the center of the top of your head. Imagine a small circle or sunburst of light there.

You may simply count your breaths as you imagine the light growing and expanding from your body into the air around you.

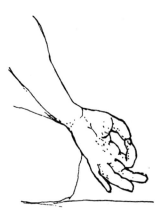

Seventh Chakra Stretch Tips

- Breathe normally as you move. Do not hold your breath.

- Flexibility increases if you do not stretch beyond your current range.

- Pain is a sign that you are out of balance.

- Slow and regular stretching gives the best results.

- Notice how when you change your exercise attitude to a more relaxed and positive one, the stretching is easier.

- Remember the Rush Reverse (see p. 36): reverse stretching can be applied to any movement, small and simple or long and complex. Choose whichever motion you want to improve and *decrease* the intensity and speed, performing it three times, doing less stretch by half each time until you can barely feel you are moving. Hold each of the three positions no longer than two seconds. Then repeat your first, largest motion range to see if your flexibility has increased.

Aromatherapy

Aromatherapy essential oils especially beneficial to the seventh chakra area include citronella, East Indian sandalwood, vetiver, patchouli, frankincense, lavender vera, and lemon balm. Used in spiritual rituals for thousands of years, frankincense slows the breathing when inhaled and thus is conducive to meditation and prayer. When applied to the skin, frankincense oil relieves dryness and scarring. The scent tends to have a calming effect, relieving anxiety and nervous tension.

Arabian mosques constructed with musk-perfumed mortar a thousand years ago still give off the scent when heated by the sun.

Seventh Chakra Stretches

WALL PRESS

This standing exercise to improve your spinal alignment is a variation of other back-flattening exercises done lying down.

1. Place your buttocks, heels, shoulders, and head against a wall.

2. Press your whole spine, from your lower back to your neck, backward. See if you can flatten against the wall. Press your spine back for two seconds as you exhale.

3. Inhale as you release. Repeat sequence several times.

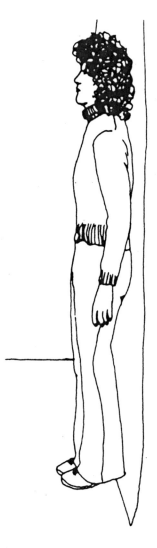

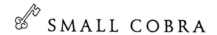 SMALL COBRA

This exercise will help release and strengthen your neck muscles.

1. Lie on your stomach on the floor. If you like, you can place a small pillow under your waist so that your back doesn't arch. Bend your elbows and place your hands, palms down, under your chin.

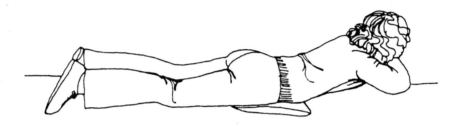

2. Lift your neck, head, and upper chest off the ground, using your lower back and stomach muscles to lift. Look up toward the ceiling as you raise your neck and upper chest as high as you comfortably can. Hold that position for a few seconds.

3. Relax your chest, then your neck, then your head down to the floor again.

4. Depending on your condition, you can also do this exercise with your hands clasped behind your head instead of on the floor.

The exercise just described is a simplified version of the full Cobra, a yoga posture in which you lift your whole torso off the ground barely using your arm muscles. You inhale as you arch and lift your torso and exhale as you come back to the ground. Don't start to do the full Cobra until your back and neck have been strengthened by doing more limited arches.

LILY

Try the Lily for a full back, leg, and neck stretch.

1. Sit on the floor with your knees bent and the soles of your feet pressed together in front of you. Hold your toes in both palms.

2. Inhale as you straighten and then arch your back. Exhale as you lean forward over your legs. Bend more at the waist than at the shoulders. Allow your head to relax toward your toes. Breathe quietly in this position. Unfold slowly.

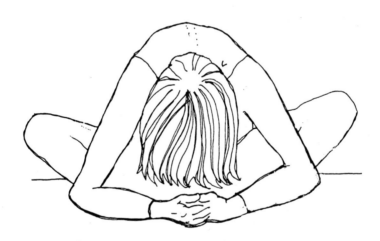

⚿ LOTUS MEDITATION

In mythology, the lotus flower represents magnificence rising from mire because its roots are in the mud but the head of the blossom always reaches up for the sun, thus making it a symbol of spiritual enlightenment. With your eyes closed, try visualizing your spine as the stalk of the plant and the top of your head as the lotus flower. Count your breaths. Imagine any physical or emotional discomfort easing away each time you exhale. Think of all your physical efforts blooming into a flexible, relaxed body and of your spirit as a lotus growing in the sun.

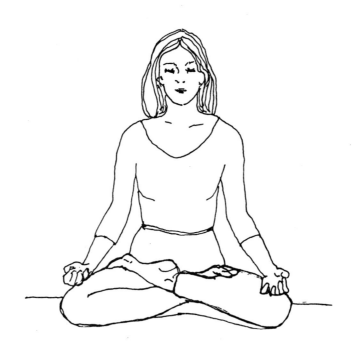

About Headaches and Exercise

Because your spine functions as a whole, constriction of the neck muscles is not the only form of tension that causes headache pain. Tension from tight shoulders, tense upper back muscles, a tilted pelvis, or constricted lower back muscles can work its way up the spine and manifest itself as a splitting headache. Approximately 20 million Americans suffer from chronic headaches and spend about 300 million dollars a year on headache medicine. For the three main types of headaches, massage or exercise can be an effective pain-relief treatment in about half the cases. When you do any exercises, be especially aware of relaxing your neck muscles. The exercises in chakras six and seven will help relieve a headache, but some of them will focus more on your individual problem areas. Experiment to see which ones reach the muscles in your body whose constriction is usually responsible for your individual tension headaches. Do your selected neck and back exercises as soon as you feel the beginnings of headache tension. This will prevent the constriction from progressing into full-blown pain. Remember to keep your neck aligned with your spine to avoid neck strain while standing or sitting.

DOUBLE BACK REST

Resting alone is healing and pleasurable. Resting with a partner can give you a jump start because relaxation can be contagious.

1. Sit on your knees back to back with toes touching. One person leans forward to rest the chest on the thighs and the forehead on the floor.

2. The other person leans back to assume a modified Fish pose, arching over his/her partner's back. If comfortable, the second person can rest his/her back and head on the partner's back.

3. Find positions without talking so you can relax and rest together. Hold the pose for a while and breathe normally.

4. Nonverbally communicate readiness to move so that the person who was curled up can now stretch back. Switch poses. Use this stretch throughout your double workout whenever you need to take a breather.

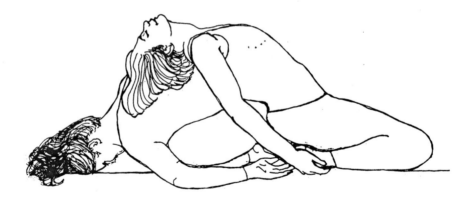

THANKS FOR THE FLEXIBILITY

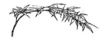

The generous flexibility exhibited by several key people in aiding the process of this book made its production possible and more enjoyable. Warm appreciation goes to my agent, Katinka Matson of Brockman, Inc.; to my editors, Claire Smith and Terry Adams, and the others, including Sarah Brennan, at Little, Brown, who were patiently encouraging; to Deborah Baker, who originally requested the project; to my typist, Suzanne Barnhill; to Ruth Morrison and Dawn Radtke, for kindly extending themselves; to my invaluable close friends, who cheered me on; to my mother and father; and to my three dogs, who were patient when their daily walks were forsaken for indoor hours by my desk.

ABOUT THE AUTHOR

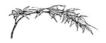

Anne Kent Rush has been practicing and writing about bodywork and alternative health care for more than thirty years, with fourteen books, including several bestsellers, to her credit. Rush has illustrated many of her own books as well those of other authors, including *The Listening Hand,* by Ilana Rubenfeld (Bantam); *The Tassajara Bread Book,* by Edward Brown (Shambhala); and *The Massage Book,* by George Downing (Random House). Rush taught on the staff of Esalen Institute, helped found Alyssum Therapy Center, and codirected Moon Books Publishers in San Francisco. Rush is also a published songwriter.

Rush has formulated a signature massage oil for the family-owned natural perfume maker Hové Parfumeur Ltd. of Louisiana. The almond-and-coconut-based oils are available online in your choice of their fresh herb and flower scents, or you can sniff test the fragrances in the eighteenth-century shop in New Orleans's French Quarter.

Printed in the United States
142494LV00003B/26/P

9 780316 172318